# PEER REVIEW
## IN
# NURSING

## PRINCIPLES FOR
## SUCCESSFUL PRACTICE

**Barbara Haag-Heitman, PhD, RN, PHCNS, BC**
Whitefish Bay, Wisconsin

**Vicki George, PhD, RN, FAAN**
Freeman, New Hampshire

**JONES AND BARTLETT PUBLISHERS**
*Sudbury, Massachusetts*
BOSTON     TORONTO     LONDON     SINGAPORE

*World Headquarters*

Jones and Bartlett Publishers
40 Tall Pine Drive
Sudbury, MA 01776
978-443-5000
info@jbpub.com
www.jbpub.com

Jones and Bartlett Publishers
Canada
6339 Ormindale Way
Mississauga, Ontario L5V 1J2
Canada

Jones and Bartlett Publishers
International
Barb House, Barb Mews
London W6 7PA
United Kingdom

Jones and Bartlett's books and products are available through most bookstores and online booksellers. To contact Jones and Bartlett Publishers directly, call 800-832-0034, fax 978-443-8000, or visit our website, www.jbpub.com.

Substantial discounts on bulk quantities of Jones and Bartlett's publications are available to corporations, professional associations, and other qualified organizations. For details and specific discount information, contact the special sales department at Jones and Bartlett via the above contact information or send an email to specialsales@jbpub.com.

# Table of Contents

# Foreword

In a postdigital world, the assurance and validation of clinical expertise and competence will become more critical and also more difficult to do. As care services increase in pace and portability, the value of establishing the relationship between process and outcome will accelerate considerably. Few tools currently exist which successfully connect these two elements of clinical effectiveness and provider competence. However, as we move more assertively into a value-driven clinical equation, a strong relationship between effectiveness and competence must become well established.

Aligning cost and contribution as a value is beyond debate. What is more difficult to accomplish is the establishment of a definitive framework within which the interaction between the two can be well established and positively advanced. The demands and the utility of evidence-based practice reflects the desire to use contemporary digital capacity as a vehicle for more strongly establishing a data-driven relationship between action and outcome. Increasingly, the possibility of both establishing and enumerating that relationship forms a good portion of the underpinning of the dynamics and practices associated with evidence-based practice. Evidentiary dynamics is grounded in the value equation. The ability to establish a rationale between actions chosen and the impact and value of those actions is critical to meaningful and sustainable clinical practice.

And yet, both the tools and the practices associated with value-driven processes are rudimentary and elemental at best. Much of our thinking and rituals related to clinical practice are still grounded in iterative and reductionistic mental models. Evidentiary dynamics, on the other hand, is firmly grounded in complexity and reflects more quantum characteristics, which move us beyond linear notions of practice and quality. In addition, ownership of one's practice and the outcomes it achieves is critical to obtaining and sustaining those outcomes and their attendant values. In the traditional hierarchic and employee-driven work model that has for generations constrained professional development and real accountability, a barrier exists that naturally limits professional accountability, which is primarily dependent on the existence and exercise of individual ownership of practice and work. Absent that ownership, both accountability and its outcomes can neither be continuously obtained nor sustained.

This fact has certainly failed to impede organizations from building rigid control structures, hierarchies, and employee-characterized work models that inherently impede the exercise of professional accountability and virtually guarantee the elimination of the necessary ownership of practice essential to both obtaining and sustaining quality outcomes. The last three decades of work on professional shared governance have more than adequately demonstrated that, if the structures of professional practice, staff-driven decision making, point-of-service accountability, and effective peer processes are absent from the organization, so also will be professional accountability, ownership, engagement, and sustainable professional practice outcomes. For professionals, it is impossible to deliver a quality you do not own, nor sustain an outcome you do not drive.

Yet, in hospitals it is quite common to divorce the ownership of quality from those who deliver it. Large offices and departments of quality exist with the sole purpose of advancing the quality of organizations and the evidence of it in their clinical work and outcomes. The problem has been and continues to be that such offices can neither drive quality nor obtain it over the long term. As Deming demonstrated decades ago: You cannot deliver a quality you do not own and you cannot manage a quality you do not deliver (1990). Now, providers have so many advisers, experts, tools, and methods, that much of the work of professional practice is now directed to advancing "scores" rather than actually making a difference in the patient's experience and in the quality of their clinical outcomes. What has happened in the majority of these health organizations is that quality has become an incremental process of data management, and the relationship and personalization necessary to both drive and sustain it has now been lost and permanently buried in the wide variety of templates, dashboards, scoreboards, charts, and other instrumentation. The means have now become the ends and the ends have become buried by the means.

Reengagement and ownership of the quality of one's work is the centerpiece of both obtaining and sustaining the quality and value of that work. The once- or twice-removed locus of control governing policy and practice of clinical care must once again be returned to the provider and be deeply indebted in the essential elements of practice and relationships between provider and patient. The locus of control for issues of practice, quality, and outcomes must be specifically located at the point of service and in the hands of those who provide that service. This direct linkage between provider and value is essential to develop the necessary ownership and engagement that is a key requisite for obtaining quality outcomes and value. Both structures and processes must converge to create the organizational circumstances and the practice obligations necessary to build the relationships and interactions essential to the delivery of high-quality practice.

It is with this understanding and in this spirit that the authors have undertaken this work on peer review. Reflecting both the principles and the evidence related to the essentials of professional practice, these authors have built a framework for practice-driven standard setting and decision making related to competence, practice, quality, and clinical outcomes. Indeed, this text focuses on creating both a frame for professional practice and models that demonstrate effectiveness and efficacy of practice driven relationships, interactions, and methods as they impact both competence and quality.

The principles and practices outlined in this text exemplify the translation of the principles of professional practice and of the shared governance structures that frame it. The authors recognize both the value of the historic experience related to the development of professional nursing practice and contemporary realities and bring that connection today in validating the appropriateness and timeliness of equity and value-based peer practices. Included are useful principles, models, and approaches to developing the kind of peer practices that demonstrate professional staff ownership of practice, competence, and quality. Furthermore, they connect this level of professional ownership to advancing both professional relationships and patient outcomes, which are the direct beneficiaries of effective peer processes.

A text such as this is long overdue. Peer processes are a fundamental element of all professional practice. Effective equity-based peer practices reflect a potential for the best that can be found and obtained from professionals embedded in their accountability, reflected in their relationship, and evidenced in their outcomes. I think you will agree. My final challenge to the reader and the user of this text is that, as you apply its principles and demonstrate real peer effectiveness, you too will share your experiences and knowledge as a part of a more generalized commitment to advancing the profession and to deepen the impact it has on those we serve.

*Tim Porter-O'Grady*

**REFERENCE**

Deming, W. E. (1990). *Total quality management.* New York, NY: Warner Books.

# Acknowledgments

Both authors would like to express their gratitude to Tim Porter-O'Grady, a fellow nurse that believes in the power of nursing and has offered endless support and guidance to our careers and this book.

## Vicki George

There are few times in your life when you are given the opportunity to reflect and pay homage to those who have made a difference in influencing your life and your life's work. First, I want to thank my family, Al, Brett, Ashleigh, and Sean, for allowing me the many hours away to explore and experience my role as a professional nurse. I want to dedicate my work here to my sister and best friend Lori, who taught me the most about nursing as she was a survivor of several chronic illnesses over the course of 20 years. Her insights were many and powerful. As Lori lay dying, she made me promise to write this book on peer review. She loved her nurses, but still at times she recognized where they could do better and be happier with their care. She wanted them to appreciate the good in each other, to help each other grow through mutual respect, and to feel the pride of their contributions to the patient's experience.

## Barb Haag-Heitman

Nothing is accomplished alone or without the tremendous support of others near and far. I am grateful for nurses from across the globe that verbalized the necessity and significance of creating this work, some who contributed their best practices included in the book. Further inspiration came from my family, Tim, Sara, and Becky, who mindfully pursue excellence in their own careers and unselfishly continually create the space for my work.

# Contributing Authors

**Kathleen Bradley, RN, MSN, NE-BC**
Director of Professional Resources
Porter Adventist Hospital
Denver, Colorado

**Paula Carynski, MS, RN, NEA-BC**
Vice President Patient Care Services
Chief Nursing Officer
OSF Saint Anthony Medical Center
Rockford, Illinois

**Gail Fyke, MSN, RN**
Decatur Memorial Hospital
Decatur, Illinois

**Nicole Jones, MN**
East Jefferson General Hospital
Metairie, Los Angeles, California

**Beth Lacoste, MSN**
East Jefferson General Hospital
Metairie, Los Angeles, California

**Timothy Porter-O'Grady, EdD, PhD, FAAN**
Senior Partner
Tim Porter-O'Grady Associates, Inc.
Atlanta, Georgia

**Dianne Forbes Woods, RN, MA, NE-C**
Deputy Nursing Director
SUNY Downstate Medical Center
Brooklyn, New York

# CHAPTER 1

# Peer Review—What It Is and What It Is Not

*Nobody can go back and start a new beginning,*
*but anyone can start today and make a new ending.*

—Maria Robinson

Insuring practitioner competency and professionalizing the discipline of nursing has been on the forefront of American nurse leaders as far back as 1896, when the American Nurses Association (ANA) was founded. Since this time, the ANA has had significant impact on the professional development of nurses and the quality of nursing care. Peer review is the essential component of professional nursing practice that helps ensure the quality and safety of care and the care provider. Unfortunately, meaningful peer review in nursing is missing in most practice environments to the detriment of both the patient and the profession.

This book advances the professional ideals of our early nurse leaders by providing guidance for the development and implementation of sustainable peer review processes. Until nursing develops and implements significant peer review processes, nursing will not achieve high levels of quality and safety outcomes for patients, clients, and society. More than 20 years have passed since the first publication of nursing guidelines for peer review, yet no organization has demonstrated full implementation of the guidelines. Also missing is the research that supports the effectiveness of current peer review practices. There is also a scarce amount of literature on effective structures, processes, and guidelines to help the practitioner implement a peer review program. This publication provides a historic look at the development of peer review and presents peer review structures and processes that will help individual nurses and healthcare organizations accomplish the quality and safety outcomes that are entrusted to them.

## THE EARLY YEARS OF PEER REVIEW

More than 35 years ago, the ANA identified peer review as a necessary part of professional nursing practice and promoted it in 1973 with the release of guidelines for the establishment of peer review committees (Flanagan, 1976). These early nurse ANA leaders declared that "the responsibility and accountability for the quality of nursing care is an integral part of each nurses' practice" (Flanagan, 1976, p. 227).

Rosamond Gabrielson served as 23rd president of the ANA from 1972 to 1976, during the time that this pioneering work in peer review was done. In her address to the Fiftieth Annual Convention on June 6, 1976, she summarized the essential professional elements necessary to advance the profession within the social content of the time. It is noteworthy that she linked peer review with quality. Her words are as applicable today as they were then.

> In the last five years, ANA has concentrated its efforts on developing tools which will assure continued quality nursing services in light of changes in nursing practice and in light of changing consumer demands. Standards of nursing practice, nursing service, and nursing education; guidelines for continuing education programming; a program for certification for excellence in clinical practice; definition of various nursing roles; and guidelines for the establishment of peer review committees are all measures aimed at judging and improving the quality of nursing performance. (Flanagan, 1976, p. 602)

The focus on peer review continued and resulted in the first publication of an ANA brochure titled, *Peer Review in Nursing Practice*, in 1983. The original, and most current, peer review guidelines came out several years later as the 1988 *Peer Review Guidelines*. Remarkably, these foundational guidelines are still pertinent today and are applicable in all professional practice environments. Tragically, the wisdom of these early nurse leaders in recognizing peer review as an essential element of ensuring nursing quality, has been overlooked in most professional practice environments to date. Most nurses seem unaware of their obligation to be involved in peer review as defined by the 1988 guidelines. The 1988 publication is now out of print and the majority of nurses educated and practicing today have not seen them, let alone integrated them into their practice. Fortunately, the American Nurses Credentialing Center (ANCC) Magnet program is helping revitalize the concept of peer review, along with other foundational elements of professional nursing practice such as autonomy (ANCC, 2005 & 2008).

Accordingly, portions of the 1988 *Peer Review Guidelines* are presented here in this chapter as an introduction to the foundational components for peer review practices that are further developed in subsequent chapters. A complete reprint of the 1988 *Peer Review Guidelines* can be found in Appendix A and should be required reading for every professional nurse.

## THE ANA *PEER REVIEW GUIDELINES*

The first section of the ANA *Peer Review Guidelines* (1988) illustrates the essential component that peer review plays in quality assurance systems for nurses at all levels and in all settings.

Peer Review Guidelines is intended to help organizational units, state nurses' associations, and individual nurses establish peer review programs. As the professional association for nursing, ANA has a responsibility to the public and its members to facilitate the development of a quality assurance system including peer review. (p. 2)

The American Nurses' Association believes nurses bear primary responsibility and accountability for the quality of nursing care their clients receive. Standards of nursing practice provide a means for measuring the quality of nursing care a client receives. Each nurse is responsible for interpreting and implementing the standards of nursing practice. Likewise, each nurse must participate with other nurses in the decision-making process for evaluating nursing care. This process is peer review.

Peer review implies that the nursing care delivered by a group of nurses or an individual nurse is evaluated by individuals of the same rank or standing according to established standards of practice. The goals of every agency providing nursing care should include peer review as one means of maintaining standards of nursing practice and upgrading nursing care. In every health care facility in which nurses practice and for each nurse in individual practice, provision for peer review should be an ongoing process. (p. 3)

The next section provides specific direction that peer review needs to be a formal process that uses professional standards as the peer review criteria. Notice that the focus on quality remains paramount.

ANA Definition of Peer Review
The generally accepted definition of peer review is an organized effort whereby practicing professionals review the quality and appropriateness of services ordered or performed by their professional peers. Peer review in nursing is the process by which practicing registered nurses systematically access, monitor, and make judgments about the quality of nursing care provided by peers as measured against professional standards of practice.

Purposes and Benefits of Peer Review
Peer review's primary focus is the quality of nursing practice. However, quality, quantity, and the cost of care are closely related: what happens in one of these

dimensions affects the two other dimensions. Quality control therefore includes attention to the related quality of care (manpower utilization) and to cost control, so patients receive only the care they need, provided at an affordable cost compatible with quality. The intent is to provide the highest quality of care at a reasonable cost. However great the external pressures for utilization and cost controls may be, the responsibility for safeguarding the quality of care is paramount. (p. 4)

The multiple purposes and benefits of peer review are then defined along with the directive that formal processes be identified and used by all nurses. Note that the ANCC Magnet Program (2008) emphasizes these aspects in their criteria requiring that nurses at all levels routinely use peer review for the assurance of competency and professional development.

The purposes of peer review are: (a) to evaluate the quality and quantity of nursing care as it is defined by the individual practitioner or a group of practitioners; (b) to determine the strengths and weaknesses of nursing care, taking into consideration local and institutional resources and constraints; (c) to provide evidence for use as the basis of recommendations for new or altered policies and procedures to improve nursing care; and (d) to identify those areas where practice patterns indicate more knowledge is needed.

Peer review activities are focused on the practice decisions of professional nurses to determine the appropriateness and timeliness of those decisions. The services provided as a result of practice decisions are also reviewed to determine their necessity, effectiveness, and efficiency.

Although informal peer review occurs whenever one nurse judiciously commends or critiques while assisting another in the management of care, the goals of nursing are best served as a formal process. Formal review includes, for example, the evaluation within the quality assurance system of an institution or an agency, and the review necessary for third party reimbursement for services provided by an individual or group of nurses. An organized program makes peer review timely and objective. Peer review can occur at various levels and situations, including in primary practice, in an institution or agency, and at the local, regional, or national level.

Individuals, institutions, and the nursing profession all derive benefits from an effective peer review program. With respect to the individual, participation in the peer review process stimulates professional growth. Clinical knowledge and skills are updated. Within the institution, effective peer review points towards changes in educational and administrative patterns needed to ensure quality, and it reveals opportunities for research pertinent to the enhancement of practice. As to the profession as a whole, improved quality of care by individuals and agencies, accompanied by self-regulation of nursing practice, can only serve to strengthen nursing.

Education of nurses on the need for and value and benefits of peer review is essential. Consideration of the following benefits may encourage the individual nurse to participate in peer review and to promote its establishment in the work environment and in the professional association.

Peer review –

- assures the consumer of the nurse's continued competence.
- provides an avenue for arbitration of consumer complaints, and complements risk-management programs by reducing the risk of suits.
- legally protects the competent nurse from unjust professional misconduct charges by providing documentation of the safety, competency, and expertness of the nurse's practice.
- rewards competent practice when data from peer review are incorporated into the performance appraisal and merit evaluations.
- identifies generic weaknesses in practice that can guide planning for staff development and continuing education programs, and new or revised policies or procedures to improve nursing care.
- increases nurses' control over nursing practice, protecting the profession from external controls and impingement by persons outside nursing.
- helps nurses fulfill the requirement in the Code for Nurses on maintaining competency in nursing.
- provides a quality assurance mechanism and documentation for health care issuers.
- assists nurses in improving documentation, communication, and productivity. (p. 5)

Thus the *Peer Review Guidelines* from 1988 provides a solid foundation for the development and implementation of contemporary peer review processes. One must acknowledge that peer review alone will not bring about the professional results and quality outcomes associated with the nursing role. Peer review is interrelated and interdependent with other components of professional practice and must occur in a professional practice environment. One cannot expect professional results from our traditional, hierarchic management of organizations. Self-regulation in professional practice environments demands that shared governance structures are in place for shared decision making and shared leadership to occur. These concepts are explored in more depth in other chapters.

## PEER REVIEW—THE TIME HAS COME

There is increasing awareness that a majority of US hospitals have significant safety and efficiency deficits (Wojcik, 2009). These concerns remain even after years of scrutiny and recommendations from organizations such as The Joint Commission, the Institute of Medicine, and the Agency for Healthcare Research and Quality.

The peer review processes in nursing recognizes that, in a self-regulating professional practice model, the clinical accountability for care rests solely with the clinical practicing nurse. It is the clinical nurse who maintains accountability for clinical practice standards, advocates for quality and safety care, ensures peer credentialing and ongoing peer review for privileging, and promotes professional development of peers within a just culture and learning environment. Clinical nurses can no longer ignore the essential role that nursing peer review plays in improving quality and safety for the clients we serve. The time is now for the entire discipline of nursing to take effective action and create meaningful structures and processes to develop peer review standards that are grounded in evidence-based practice, the novice to expert continuum, and the day-to-day, shift-to-shift focus on improving patient outcomes. This work is what the public entrusts nursing to deliver.

Quality in performance and self-regulation of the discipline are hallmarks of a mature profession. Peer review is the mechanism by which the profession holds itself accountable to society. Therefore, a national call to action around nursing peer review is essential. The only focused action regarding peer review at this time is located in the ANCC Magnet program. The Magnet program highlights peer review as one of the foundational elements of professional practice and professional practice environments (ANCC, 2008). Peer review for nurses at all levels and in all settings of the organization is necessary to achieve Magnet designation (ANCC, 2008). No organization has completely implemented the ANA guidelines or achieved the outcomes as just described. In addition, no best practice framework has been established.

## THE ROLE OF THE MANAGEMENT IN PEER REVIEW

In our experience, many organizations are under the misconception that peer review is a managerial process performed at the time of the annual performance review. Peer review is not a managerial accountability. Many organizations are confused about the role of the manager in peer review. Positioning managers to take the lead on peer review processes violates the definition for clinical nurse peers as illustrated in the 1988 *Guidelines for Peer Review*. In addition, the annual performance review lacks the dynamic real-time practice feedback necessary to focus the practitioner on the achievement of everyday excellence in quality and safety outcomes. Additionally, the conventional use of anonymous staff input into the annual performance review of their peers leaves the recipient without the ability to gain insight into the feedback from others to enhance their personal and professional growth. Anonymity violates the principles of skilled communication as defined in the American Association of Critical-Care Nurses' *Healthy Workplace Environment Initiative* (Barden, 2005). Unfortunately, this process of anonymous staff input has tarnished the notion of peer review for many. Nurses also report a lack of training for giving and receiving feedback as well as a fear of retaliation as barriers to giving honest feedback. This deficit often results in a lack of constructive feedback and many times the giving of inflated affirming feedback with no behavioral change. Some coin the ineffective process "pal" review, further contributing to the negative connotation that many nurses currently have about the peer review process, and contributing to a lack of productivity and wasteful efforts.

The manager's role in peer review is to support the peer review processes by providing the necessary resources to ensure a supportive practice environment for the clinical nurse to practice, to engage in quality and safety initiatives, and to develop professionally. In a report on employee engagement and labor relations, the manager's role is to align the organization and remove systematic barriers (Tyler, 2009). Managers must be sure that what is recognized and rewarded is encouraged and sustainable in the organization, including peer review. By constantly identifying and eliminating barriers to high performance in professional processes such as peer review, the manager promotes an engaged and productive culture. Eliminating barriers such as lack of information, poor communication skills, poor technology, and inequity in compensation at the time of performance evaluation are managerial responsibilities.

## THE ROLE OF NURSING EDUCATION IN PEER REVIEW

Nursing education should partner with management to provide the educational framework to foster an ongoing learning environment and help eliminate these barriers to peer review. The measurement of clinical competencies for clinical nurses in all settings is well understood in nursing education. The development and measurement of the following competencies should be treated in the same way as clinical competencies. These competencies include how to interpret quality data; shared leadership skills, including challenging the status quo and leading the way; communication skills including negotiation, facilitation, and conflict management; and professional role actualization and peer review principles. These new competencies need to be assessed and measured in the same way as clinical competencies have been in the past. These competencies need to be included in the orientation and ongoing professional development of the nurse.

## THE ROLE OF NURSING SERVICE AND ACADEMIC PARTNERSHIPS IN PEER REVIEW

It is essential that leadership competencies be incorporated into the undergraduate curriculum for all nurses. Situating this educational process at the very beginning of the novice's learning will enculturate the nurse into the professional processes of leading and developing effective peer review systems. By setting new expectations for performance around leadership, role actualization, and peer review participation, a new generation of nurses will have the skills necessary to lead the cultural transformation. Removing the negative connotations around peer review will take inspirational leaders to transform the culture and create the positive professional image of peer review linked to improving healthcare outcomes.

## PEER REVIEW—THE TIME IS NOW

The vision that early nursing leaders had for a robust peer review process to achieve quality patient outcomes has not been realized. Regular peer feedback on the performance of nursing care would seems all but lost if not for the peer review concepts that are described in the best practice models throughout the text. However, no organization has implemented all the elements of the conceptual model described in this primer.

The time is now for nursing leaders and direct care practitioners to collaborate and embrace peer review as a professional mandate for improving patient quality and safety. The latest report from the Centers for Medicare and Medicaid Services (CMS) indicates that the rate of medical errors is actually increasing and the death toll from preventive medical injuries approaches 200,000 per year in the United States. (Crowley & Hearst, 2009). Nursing must define and demonstrate effectiveness at what the public and other healthcare practitioners recognize as nurses' vital role. The role of the nurse as patient advocate is to ensure patient quality and safety through recognition of early warning signs, to challenge inappropriate care, and to rescue patients from harm. From the time of Florence Nightingale, nurses have played a significant role in preventing infections in hospitalized patients, yet as recently as 2009, a study by the Centers for Disease Control and Prevention concluded that 99,000 patients succumb to hospital-acquired infections annually (Crowley & Hearst, 2009). Nursing peer review is the missing essential element needed to ensure that nurses hold each other accountable to improve these and other quality outcomes for patient care.

The purpose of this book is to revitalize nursing peer review and bring back its original focus on quality patient outcomes along with the contemporary addition of patient safety. An expansion and extension of the focus of peer review to professional role actualization and nursing practice advancement is also promoted. The book begins with the history of peer review development by the ANA. The next chapter emphasizes the tenets of being part of a profession and the professional code of ethics that accompany these principles. A conceptual framework is provided to assist all professionals in an organizational context to frame an effective peer review design. An implementation framework based on the shared governance principles of ownership, equity, partnership, and accountability provides the reference for self-regulation of the discipline. Examples of formal types of peer review structures and practices for nurses at all levels and in all settings of the organization are illustrated. These best practices of organizations will help lead the way in developing and integrating interactive models of peer review.

An informal mechanism of peer review, Targeted Improvement for Patient Safety (TIPS), is proposed for daily improvement in quality and safety. TIPS is a practical innovation to systematize an informal peer review process that happens every day as the nurses between shifts hand off the care of a team of patients. TIPS can be used to address the targeted improvement goals for quality and safety specific to the unit and the patients served. By individualizing the approach to safety with each patient, the nurse can assure patient involvement and family teaching. And lastly, the educational programming needed prior to advancing peer-to-peer feedback is presented. These shared leadership techniques are evidence based and serve to increase the level of professionalism of the staff. While developing as leaders and improving their communication methods, staff deliver a higher quality of care based on autonomy in practice (George, 1999).

This is the first nursing book on peer review, defining what it is and what it is not. Nurses are encouraged to use this primer to explore innovative ways to use peer review to improve patient quality and safety. Implementing the ANA principles of peer review will facilitate the responsibility and accountability for the quality of nursing practice to rest in the hands of the professional and not be directed by others in health care. By using the principles of peer review, the profession of nursing can be united about nursing's unique role in advocating for the highest quality health care.

## REFERENCES

American Nurses Association. (1988). *Peer review guidelines*. Kansas City, MO: Author.

American Nurses Credentialing Center. (2005). *Magnet application manual*. Silver Spring, MD: Author.

American Nurses Credentialing Center. (2008). *Application manual Magnet recognition program*. Silver Spring, MD: Author.

Barden, C. (Ed.). (2005). *AACN standards for establishing and sustaining healthy work environments*. Aliso Viejo, CA: AACN.

Crowley, C., & Hearst, E. N. (2009, August). *Within health care hides massive, avoidable death toll*. Available at: http://www.chron.com/disp/story.mpl/deadbymistake/6555095.html. Accessed on August 17, 2009.

Flanagan, L. (Ed.). (1976). *One strong voice: The story of the American Nurses' Association.* Kansas City, MO: ANA.

Tyler, J. (2009, September). Employee engagement and labor relations. *Gallup Management Journal.* Available at: http://gmj.gallup.com/content/122849/Employee-Engagement-Labor-Relations.aspx. Accessed September 11, 2009.

Wojcik, J. (2009, April). Hospitals fall short on safety, quality: Leapfrog. *Business Insurance.* Available at: http://www.businessinsurance.com/article/20090415/NEWS/200015959. Accessed April 29, 2009.

# CHAPTER 2

# Becoming a Profession

*"One has to study the old to establish the new."*

—CHINESE PROVERB

## STUDYING THE OLD: A HISTORIC AND LITERARY SYNOPSIS

Nursing has not always been considered a true profession in the United States. In the early part of the 19th century, the lack of consistent educational standards, along with an absence of an ethical code of conduct, contributed to nursing being identified as a subprofession by the US federal government. Peer review is another dimension of professionalism that was not in place at the time. Peer review is a critical defining element separating jobs from professional occupations, not only in nursing, but also in the medical field, in law, and in engineering. To maintain role autonomy and professional status, effective peer review processes that ensure quality of the provider and quality of the practice must be in place.

### Understanding the Old

The history of nursing in the United States is marked by landmark decisions and actions that have brought about nursing as we know it today. Without these key moments, nursing might still be under the control and direction of hospital committees and the medical profession as it was in the mid-1800s until the early 1920s.

The story of nursing becoming a profession in the United States and highlights of associated important political developments are chronicled in the book *One Strong Voice: The Story of the American Nurses' Association* (American Nurses Association [ANA], 1976). The story begins with the American colonies seeking independence from outside rule, mirroring how nursing would seek its independence some 150 years later.

### The Revolutionary War

One of the first political leaders of the United States was George Washington, who recognized the need for organized care for sick and wounded soldiers. Women participated in the care and were called nurses, but because formal

11

training did not yet exist, they mostly supported soldiers nutritionally and performed housekeeping duties. Washington called for legislation to establish army hospitals in the years 1775 and 1777, including a bill to establish a ratio of nurses proportionate to the number of sick and wounded soldiers (ANA, 1976). This may have been the first attempt to set nurse-to-patient ratios to ensure patient outcomes. Unfortunately, after the war, efforts to establish an effective healthcare system were neglected.

## The Civil War

The need for a trained core of nurses to care for wounded soldiers emerged again during the Civil War in 1861. Little to no progress had been made in the training of nurses since the previous national war 80 years earlier. Hospitals were still ill adapted to care for sick and wounded soldiers. Most of the nursing functions during the Civil War were carried out by women of religious orders. The need for an organized workforce of nursing, as identified by George Washington decades earlier, became part of the national agenda again (ANA, 1976).

## The Influence of Florence Nightingale on Nursing Education

Around this same time, Florence Nightingale was establishing the first nursing training schools in England following the Crimean War. Medical leaders in the United States noticed that British nurses trained under Nightingale contributed to a decrease in mortality rates and subsequently advocated for the use of Nightingale's principles for nursing education in the United States (ANA, 1976). In 1873, the occupation of nursing was established in the United States in the public domain coinciding with the opening of the first schools of nursing. This historic event set the foundation for nursing to become a profession utilizing educational standards and a commitment to public service.

### *Nightingale Principles of Nursing Education*

Nightingale's principles on nursing education significantly impacted training schools for nursing in the United States. Her efforts support the autonomy of nursing from physicians while also identifying the interdependency and collaborative aspects. The following Nightingale principles helped set the foundation for nursing to become a profession in the years to come.

- A training school for nurses should be closely connected with hospitals but independently administered.
- Training school for nurses should be considered an educational institution and receive public funds.

- The nursing administrator must be granted the authority to act independently of the physician's disease-treatment mandate to uphold the nursing mandate for health and healing.
- Supervision of nursing training in all aspects of care should come from nursing leaders who are themselves trained and experienced.
- A professional nurse should assume the directorship of administration and take responsibility for education of the nursing students. (Dossey, Selanders, Beck, & Attewell, 2005)

Further attempts to elevate nursing to a true profession during this time came from nursing pioneer leader Abbey Woolsey, who, in 1876, stressed that the need for nursing training schools be elevated to institutions of higher education, thus enhancing the status as an educated and honorable profession (ANA, 1976). Unfortunately, the public did not recognize the need for public funding of nursing schools. Schools that did try to remain independent of hospitals eventually closed because of financial hardships. Those that remained open ultimately became incorporated as part of the hospital. Tragically, the once autonomous schools of nursing, whose responsibility was to develop the profession and to set standards and methods of education, were now run by hospital administrators who determined that nursing education and skill development would be placed under the authority of the medical staff. Nursing became a by-product of service to the institution, rather than in service to the public as previously defined by the Nightingale principles.

## Establishment of ANA

Although the establishment of nursing schools as described previously helped produce an adequate quantity of nurses in the United States, measures of quality and competence still need to be addressed. Early nurse leaders did not lose sight of these professional mandates and continued to pursue means for nursing to develop into its own independent profession. This interest in advancing nursing educationally and professionally led to the establishment of the ANA in 1896. Throughout the early history of nursing in America, the profession labored over three major concerns:

1. The need to develop criteria based on educational preparation and practical experience to determine competency.
2. The need to establish laws that set forth standards for nurses to function in a professional capacity.
3. The need to create descriptive terminology that reflected nursing functions and levels of competency. (ANA, 1976)

**Establishing Professional Status**

Issues related to education preparation for nursing became a barrier to achieving professional status. Other professional elements, including a code of ethics and peer review for competency assurance, also needed to be addressed. During this time of ANA's formulation, nurse leader Isabel Hampton Robb pointed out that, collectively, nursing could not qualify as a profession because it lacked many of the criteria used during the time to define professionals (ANA, 1976).

The professional criteria at the time came from the work of Dr. Abraham Flexner. In 1910, Dr. Flexner defined the following characteristics of a profession:

1. A profession involves a high degree of individual responsibility.
2. A profession professes a body of specialized knowledge and skill.
3. A profession aims to provide practical and definite service.
4. A profession is characterized by self-organization and self-regulation.
5. A profession's motivation tends to be altruistic. (ANA, 1976, p. 23)

With these criteria in hand, pioneering nurse leaders of the ANA set about to establish nursing as a full profession by taking control of nursing educational programs regulation and standards of practice development, and by establishing ways to measure practitioner competency. The first challenge to the ANA's control of nursing practice was during the period between 1924 and 1934. The federal government established a Personnel Classification Board as a result of the 67th US Congress, whose purpose was to establish a set of determinants that would categorize professional from nonprofessional workers in government service. The bill outlined that educational preparation of the practitioner would be used as criteria for determination of a profession. The educational requirements included professional, scientific, or technical training equivalent to graduation from a college or university.

Using these criteria, a decision was made in 1924 by the government that because of the lack of consistency in nursing education, nursing was deemed to be in the nonprofessional category. At the time, nursing education varied from an eighth grade preparation to a university degree. In response, much effort went into defining educational preparation of nurses using collaborate efforts of many nursing and nonnursing organizations.

**Establishing Ethical Standards**

Another missing professional element for nursing was a code of conduct based on ethical principles. In response, the ANA Committee on Ethical Standards was formed to develop a statement of ideals, rather than simply outlining good conduct. During the 1926 ANA convention, these ideals were approved and set the stage for the elements of modern day nursing. In addition, these ethical statements became the framework for the profession and how each professional nurse should conduct his or her practice. These elements are listed below as the ANA Ethical Standards of Nursing from 1926 (ANA, 1976). The purpose of the standards was not to be specific as it related to individual practice situations, but to provide an ethical framework from which all other standards might flow.

*The Relation of the Nurse to the Patient:*
The nurse should bring to the care of the patient all of the knowledge, skill and devotion which she may posses. To do this she must appreciate the relationship of the patient to his family and to his community. The nurse must broaden her thoughtful consideration of the patient to include family, friends, for only in surroundings that are harmonious and peaceful can the nurse give her utmost skill, devotion and knowledge to safeguard the health of patient and protection of property.

*The Relation of the Nurse to the Medical Profession:*
The term "medicine" should be understood to relate to *scientific* medicine and the desirable relationship between the two should be one of mutual respect. The nurse should be fully informed of the provisions of the medical practice of her own state in order than she may not unconsciously support malpractice or infringement of the law. The key to the situation lies in the mutuality of aim of medicine and nursing: to cure and prevent disease and promote positive health; the techniques are different and neither profession can secure complete results without the other.

*The Relation of the Nurse to the Allied Professions:*
The health of the public has come to demand many services other than nursing. Without the closest interrelation of workers and appreciation of the ethical standards of all groups and a clear understanding of the limitations of her own group, the best results in building positive health in the community cannot be obtained.

*Relation of Nurse to Nurse:*
The "Golden Rule" embodies all that could be written in many pages on the relation of nurse to nurse. This should be one of fine loyalty, of appreciation for work conscientiously done, and respect for positions of authority. On the other hand, loyalty to the motive which inspires nursing as a profession should make the nurse fearless to bring to light any serious violations to the ideals herein expressed. The larger loyalty is that to the common good, to the community, for this loyalty to an ideal is larger than any personal loyalty.

*Relation of the Nurse to Her Profession:*
The nurse has a definite responsibility to her profession as a whole. The contribution of individual service is not enough. She should, in addition, give reasonable portion of her time to the furtherance of such advancements of the profession

as are only possible through action of the group as a whole. This involves attendance at meetings and the acquisition of information, for intelligent participation in such matters as organizational and legislation decisions. The supreme responsibility of the nurse in relation to her profession is to keep the spiritual flame which has illuminated the work of great nurses of all time. (ANA, 1976, pp. 89–91)

### Establishing the Role of the Professional Nurse

When, in 1930, the Personnel Classification Board announced its decision to place nursing in the category of subprofessional workers, the ANA used both the Flexner report and the Nursing Standards of Ethical Practice to formulate the following definitions of nursing and the role of the professional nurse that was adopted by the delegation the following year.

> Professional Nursing. Professional nursing is a blend of intellectual attainments, attitudes and manual skills based on the principles of scientific medicine, acquired by means of a prescribed course in a school of nursing affiliated with a hospital, recognized for such purposes by the state and practiced in conjunction with curative or preventive medicine, by the individual licensed to do so by the state.
>
> Professional Nurse. Therefore, a professional nurse is one who has met all the legal requirements for registration in a state and who practices or holds a position by virtue of her professional knowledge and legal status. (ANA, 1976, p. 92)

As the ANA began to grow in membership, its role in advocating for legislation that would impact nursing and the nursing work environments furthered. It was the ANA position that nursing practice standards should be the responsibility of each practitioner and that each practitioner should be accountable for the quality of nursing care provided.

It was at the 1972 ANA convention, responding to a House of Delegates vote in 1970 request, that ANA support methods were established through which nurses could have a definite and effective voice in their practice.

### Becoming a Profession: Establishing the New

Efforts to establish nursing with a professional status were championed by America's early nurse leaders who came together to collectively advance nursing and who formed the ANA. Using Florence Nightingale's principles, the ANA helped establish nursing educational standards, ethical standards, and definitions for professional nursing and the professional nurse. These accomplishments created the foundation for further professionalizing nursing— including defining the key role of peer review in ensuring quality care and a quality care provider.

## Defining the Need for Peer Review

During the 1972 ANA convention, delegates set forth that every healthcare facility needed a "provision for continuing peer review as one means of maintaining standards of nursing practice" (ANA, 1976, p. 226). Thus, the ANA House of Delegates charged all nurses to accept responsibility for their own involvement in quality care measures, including peer review. Subsequently, the ANA appointed an ad hoc committee to develop the first nursing peer review guidelines. The members of this ad hoc committee included representatives of the ANA's nursing congress, nursing commissions, divisions on practice, and the National Student Nurses' Association (ANA, 1976). This group became the Ad Hoc Committee on Implementation of Standards and published *Peer Review: Guidelines for Establishment of Committees*, in 1973. In this document, peer review is defined as "the process by which registered nurses, actively engaged in the practice of nursing, appraise the quality of nursing care in a given situation in accordance with established standards of practice" (ANA, 1976, p. 226). Additionally, the ad hoc committee indicated that the purposes of peer review are:

1. To evaluate the quality and the quantity of nursing care as it is delivered by the individual practitioner and/or group of practitioners, the purpose being to identify the extent of consistency to established standards of practice.
2. To determine the strengths and weakness of nursing care.
3. To provide evidence to utilize as the basis of recommendations for new or altered policies and procedures to improve nursing care.
4. To identify those areas where practice patterns indicate more knowledge is needed. (ANA, 1976, p. 226)

## Implementing the Standards of Practice

Also at the 1972 ANA convention was a resolution on the Implementation of Standards of Nursing Practice within Employment Settings declaring the "collective participation by nurses in shaping decisions that affect conditions of employment and practice is inseparable from and contributes to the goal of implementing high standards of nursing practice" (ANA, 1976, p. 225–226). A new professional organizational mode called shared governance emerged as the first attempt to implement this new direction. A professional organizational construct linked to, but separate from, the traditional hierarchic nursing administration structure was described by Dr. Timothy Porter-O'Grady in 1984 and subsequent publications described the process of self-regulation. Historically, it appears that the concepts of peer review and shared governance emerged during the same period of time and are interwoven as essential components of professional practice as described by Greenwood (1957).

**Essential Components of Professional Practice**

Building on the work of Flexner, scholars of the 1950s and 1960s added concepts derived from the work of Greenwood (1957) and others to promote nursing in an organizing professional framework. Not unlike the medical staff, professional elements of credentialing and privileging were identified along with a need for bylaws to describe the work of the discipline so other organizational partnerships could develop. The current use of these tenets or professional elements include the following:

1. Professionals must practice with a knowledge defined by the research of their discipline.
2. Professional nurses must identify with peers through an organizing structure for the purposes of applying the evidence-based practice, measuring the standards of this practice, and reporting its outcomes to the public.
3. The professional nurses must engage in a form of peer review to ensure the standards of the practitioner are met and the trust of the public is maintained in them for judgment and attention to the client's welfare.
4. The professional nurses must have a unique relationship with the client, based in the behavioral expectations of the Code of Ethics for Nursing.

**A Historic Look at Peer Review**

As a developing profession, nursing had many of these components in place, with the exception of consistent peer review processes and effective shared governance structures. As the numbers of professionals grew, there was an explosion of interest focused on nursing theory and research by the both national and international nursing communities. The unique nurse–client relationship was defined by American nurse researcher and theorist, Virginia Henderson, who defined the role of the nurse as follows: "to assist the individual, sick or well, in the performance of those activities contributing to health or its recovery (or to a peaceful death) that he would perform unaided if he had the necessary strength, will, or knowledge" (ANA, 2003, p. 68–69).

Many organizations during this time claimed to have some form of nursing shared governance structure; however, there were often deficits in terms of bylaws development and decision making authority for the discipline. Reporting relationships within the nursing management structure were changing rapidly and there was confusion around membership in the discipline. Financial and professional support in terms of protected time for shared governance participation waxed and waned according to the employment setting or the nursing management structure.

Although the publication of the first ANA guidelines for peer review occurred in 1983, the literature over the next decade is void in the application of these concepts. Unknowingly, nursing managers appeared to accept the responsibility for peer review under the context of performance evaluation, which was emerging during this time. It is important then for the purposes of this work that we define and reaffirm the tenets of professional practice in their entirety as they are the basis of all that we must do as a professional in nursing.

### Lessons Learned in Peer Review

In nursing, as in all professions, peer review is an essential part of maintaining professional control over practice, and a process that professionals use to hold themselves accountable for their services to the public, the profession, and the organization. Peer review plays an essential role in ensuring quality outcomes, fostering practice development, and maintaining professional autonomy.

The literature describes various approaches and applications of nursing peer review. Practice-related articles are often case reports on projects or processes of a single unit, or have a specialty practice focus. No whole systems approaches have been reported, creating a void and an opportunity for the profession. Rout and Roberts (2007) published a systematic review of the literature on peer review from 1994 onward, identifying ways how peer review is used in nursing. This review includes articles from the United States and five other countries. Four types of peer review emerged from this literature review: (1) projects involving staff working in practice, (2) staff working in higher education, (3) students in higher education, and (4) students in practice. Most of the literature on staff involvement came from the acute care setting versus primary care or other settings. Rout and Roberts concluded that there is a lack of robust literature on peer review. Their integrated literature review report is presented in Table 2-1. Six of the studies from this review are highlighted here as their focus; findings and subsequent lessons learned support principles for contemporary peer review process.

### Using Peer Review for Continuous Quality Improvement

One organization used a continuous quality improvement framework to create a new peer review processes for direct care nurses. Cohen, Berube, and Turrentine (1996) described the following reasons for making changes in their peer review processes:

- Feedback was often subjective rather than objective, reflecting attitudes rather than focusing on behaviors.
- There was a "Halo and Horns" phenomenon, and feedback was either wholly positive or wholly negative and therefore not considered useful or valid.
- Feedback was frequently anonymous, reflecting discomfort and fear of reprisal.

- Feedback was usually only requested by a supervisor as part of a disciplinary or promotional process.
- The feedback was often not timely, focusing on the most recent behavior, and therefore did not promote growth.
- There was no coherent feedback process.

Using this information they developed a peer review model with the following seven principles:

1. A peer is a professional nurse responsible for his or her own professional growth.
2. Peer review should promote professional growth and improve the quality of care.
3. Peer review should be timely, ongoing, and frequently done.
4. Peer review should not be connected only to performance evaluation or promotional opportunities (like clinical ladders).
5. Peer review may be formal or informal, verbal or written, but not anonymous.
6. Peer review should address specific objective behaviors in the delivery of patient care and quality.
7. Peer review should be documented.

### Lessons Learned

These authors included seven important aspects into their peer review processes. These include peer review that incorporates timely feedback, is not anonymous, promotes professional development, improves the quality of care, and targets specific objectives. The authors identified two areas for process improvement, more education of supervisors before implementation and the inclusion of more clinicians in the education process.

### Using Shared Governance to Design Peer Review

Larson and Herrick (1996) described the successful implementation of peer review and achieving targeted outcomes through integrating peer review into the professional practice model of shared governance. When the authority for practice change is vested in a shared governance structure, they described the development, implementation, and evaluation of a peer review tool within a shared governance framework. Collaboration between councils was necessary to bring about the targeted change of promoting professional development, fostering a group philosophy and a forum for recognition. The authors reported that this shared decision making framework and peer review process promotes staff ownership and accountability of the practice, and helps staff measure their own performance against expectations. A refinement of the tool was done based on staff input to make it less subjective and more accurately reflect performance according to the defined standards. To promote clarification of feedback, an open identification, nonanonymous process was implemented.

### Lessons Learned

Important principles promoted by these authors include use of defined practice standards agreed upon by the peer group, use of the shared governance structure for the decision making process, and use of a nonanonymous feedback to promote accountability and ownership to the practice review.

### Using Unit-Based Council to Implement Peer Review

Pedersen (2004) describes the development of a unit-based peer review council to evaluate performance and hold practitioners accountable to their decisions and bedside care. The peer review council adopted a philosophy that was in alignment with the hospital's mission and values that would support fairness and a humanistic approach. Feedback was targeted to address positive and growth-producing peer input. Training on giving supportive and developmental feedback was provided prior to implementation. The author reported that staff indicated support for the change.

An evaluation of the new process after one year yielded some unexpected yet positive outcomes as follows:

- Individuals and members of the Peer Review Council began to identify and address issues prior to the evaluations in order to help staff improve performance.
- Members of the council wanted the staff to excel and also wanted to prevent managerial intervention so that the staff has a chance to change behavior or performance.
- A level of comfort developed in addressing incomplete tasks or care issues with individuals.

### Lessons Learned

Peer review principles in this practice included having a defined practice focus, using peers from the same rank as the reference group to do the peer evaluation, the importance of staff ownership, using peer feedback as a routine not a static process, and staff awareness of coaching and mentoring for peer practice improvement.

### Using Student Peer Review for Role Actualization

Sedlak and Doheny (1998) identified the important role that peer review plays in promoting students' critical thinking when used in the process of student-led clinical rounds. These authors describe the following aspects of student-led clinical rounds:

- Presenting important physical and psychosocial assessment findings in a two to three minute report.
- Identifying and prioritizing pertinent nursing diagnosis, nursing interventions, and outcomes.
- Introducing the patient to peer group when possible.
- Reviewing the documentation with peers for accuracy and completeness.

The reported outcomes of the use of this student-led clinical rounds protocol include:

- Students' identification of peer review as a vehicle for developing their critical thinking and organizational skills.
- Critical thinking skills developed and new perspectives were learned as they shared their perspectives with others.
- Peer review seemed to foster self-esteem and self-confidence.
- The experience was seen as an opportunity for learning and growth in a supportive environment.
- The rounds can facilitate team interaction and enhance self-direction.

### *Lessons Learned*

The introduction of peer review as a professional practice should be part of basic nursing education. The sharing of perspective with others appears to foster self-esteem and self-confidence leading to growth of autonomy. Using face-to-face peer interaction enhances teamwork. The developmental stage of the nurse and associated expectations are important to incorporate into the peer review.

### Peer Review Education for Successful Implementation

Brooks, Olsen, Rieger-Kligys, and Mooney (1995) describe the development of a peer review process on this unit to enhance professional practice. The work began with the creation of a mission statement to guide the work; "To provide higher quality nursing practice through peer evaluations. Peer review will encompass staff accountability, clinical performance and staff commitment, thereby increasing staff cohesiveness and trust to promote team building within the shared governance framework" (p. 38).

The authors also provide insight into the importance of providing education on communication for effective peer review and to enhance the professional practice environment. Promoting and communicating each individual's practice enhances teamwork, encourages creativity, and creates a sense of ownership regarding nursing practice among all members of the team. Education in communication skills was also critical for all members. The educational sessions included listening skills practice, confrontation techniques, and strategies for giving and receiving feedback. In addition, an algorithm was developed to assist the staff with learning the methodology for addressing problems directly with each other, rather than taking issues to the managers.

### *Lessons Learned*

The role of education for communication skill development, such as giving and receiving feedback and confrontation techniques, is a key to success. Lack of effective communication skills is often reported as a barrier to peer review. The role of a mission statement is critical to creating a responsive environment.

### Peer Review for APNs

Cheyne, Niven, and McGinley (2003) researched the use of peer review to promote quality practice in the advanced practice nurse (APN) role. They described an APN case review model called PEER (peer, education, evaluation, review).

The PEER case review model established the following guidelines:

1. The clinical reviews are confidential.
2. Positive feedback and critical evaluation were to be used.
3. Each participant was a practicing midwife (a direct care practitioner of the same rank).

Prior to the study, the anticipated benefits of peer review included:

- a learning experience,
- an opportunity to review and reflect on practice,
- peer support and improved trust with colleagues,
- confidence-building and improved self-esteem, and
- an improved clinical outcome.

The anticipated problems included:

- negative criticism,
- difficulty in being completely open for fear of what others might think,
- problems with group dynamics, and
- failure to admit to mistakes.

The authors report positive outcomes, including reported changes in practice, changes in record keeping and documentation, improved practice evaluation, and problem-solving skills. Over half of the participants indicated that peer support was the best part of the process, followed by the importance of learning from each other.

## *Lessons Learned*

The APN supervisor's role in peer review was to provide support and development of an exemplary practice that was not disciplinary in nature. Practicing APNs lead the process with a supervisor participating as a member of the team. The supervisor brings expert knowledge of regulatory standards. Learning from one another can occur using peer review.

## Implications for Peer Review Development and Implementation

From a system's perspective, it is clear that no author has described a whole systems approach to peer review either in his or her clinical specialty or in his or her organizational context. These are descriptions of single unit, single role, or single specialty applications. No literature existed that described any peer review best practices for managers, directors, or the CNO.

The lessons learned support the following essential elements to be incorporated for all clinicians attempting to design and implement a peer review process. The following essential elements are articulated from the literature review:

1. The design and implementation of peer review must be done using the self-regulating structure of shared governance. Therefore, a structure of shared governance must be present at all levels and in all settings in the organization, system, and unit.
2. Adoption of the ANA peer review principles is a shared governance decision making process and becomes the foundation of the design work.
3. Peer review processes must be designed, evaluated, and used by peers of the same rank. Peer review must be in a whole system design framework and include participation by all members of the discipline, in all settings of the organization.
4. The manager must be clear on the differences between performance evaluation and disciplinary action as described in the employee handbook and the process of peer review defined in the shared governance bylaws.
5. Education about the peer review process and the skills necessary to implement the peer review work must be provided before starting the process.
6. The manager establishes the responsive environment and provides the resources for the peer review process to occur.
7. The managers and staff use coaching and mentoring skills to improve practice and build self-confidence through teamwork.
8. The methodology for feedback, both clinical and personal, should be based on objective measurable data and the standards of practice defined by the discipline.

9. Peer review encompasses timely, routine, and continuous feedback and is never an anonymous process.
10. The developmental stage of the nurse, and associated expectations, are incorporated into the peer review process.

## PROFESSIONAL PRACTICE ACCOUNTABILITY AND AUTONOMY

Peer review is not about tools, forms, or processes, but rather it is about a fundamental belief in the role actualization of a professional. It is about accepting professional accountability and autonomy in nursing practice. It is about accepting that one cannot practice autonomously without developing a measurement of accountability. The social and economic importance of ensuring high-quality patient outcomes within a rapidly shifting healthcare system calls for nursing to demonstrate autonomy in practice. Therefore, this practice autonomy forces the discipline to develop new measures of accountability and peer review.

Because nurses are by volume and by proximity the closest practitioners to the client served, it is imperative that they be charged with developing peer review processes that keep the patient safe. Advocating for high-quality outcomes from all disciplines that could add to or harm the patient in the clinical setting is the fundamental role of the nurse. It is imperative that nurses practice this high level of autonomy so they can facilitate the patient experience and achieve the best possible outcomes.

Today, these concepts sometimes appear lost to contemporary nursing education and unrecognized in today's nursing practice environment. Advancement of these tenets, and peer review in particular, requires a renewed understanding of professional autonomy and accountability. Both are discussed in more detail in the next section.

### Professional Practice Accountability

Accountability for peer review is based on the codes one subscribes to when taking on a professional role. Accountability is part of the Code of Ethics for Nurses.

As a professional, each provider is answerable to the profession and to the public for his or her professional actions, decisions, and outcomes. In addition, nurses practicing collectively are accountable for their joint outcomes. It is at this practice juncture that peer review plays an essential role in delivering patient outcomes, promoting role actualization, and advancing practice through autonomy. In a systematic way, all three must be attended to and barriers that would interfere with superior practice performance be removed. Practice performance must be measured if accountability is to exist.

**Professional Practice Autonomy**

Autonomy is another essential component of professional practice. Autonomy is the freedom to make decisions at the point of care and to choose actions without external controls (Porter-O'Grady & Finnigan, 1984). The nurse also has the right to participate in decision making that affects the discipline as a whole. Nurses, through their experiential learning, can translate that learning into new standards of care and practice. In an ever changing and challenging practice environment, this aspect of autonomy, and the professional's right to practice with new knowledge, is critical to achieving quality patient outcomes. Any constraint on the direct care nurses' autonomy can serve as a basis for conflict between direct care nurses and nursing management. Unresolved conflict emerges when there is no sustainable and identifiable structure to address these conflicts in a truly collaborative fashion. Leading to the best possible decisions, shared governance, with a formalized set of bylaws, rules, and regulations, provides the ideal and tested framework to ensure that conflict resolution occurs. Professional autonomy occurs when the discipline self-regulates and holds itself responsible. Accountability occurs when autonomy of practice is measured by peer review.

**Peer Review Within the Nursing Quality Structure**

Professional practice behaviors are based on intellect, but experientially framed. This aspect of nursing as a practice discipline requires the formation of peer review structures that facilitate this process. Newly acquired learning through experience is translated in many ways through multiple venues of collaboration. Nurses are team players in caring for patients or unique patient populations. Peer review is a process that can be used to advance the discipline by giving feedback to each individual practitioner as well as the team as a whole. Peer review is part of a quality assurance system and is best understood when placed in the context of nursing quality assurance effort (ANA, 1988). Figure 2-1 describes how peer review is positioned within a nursing quality assurance system.

**Utilizing the Quality Assurance Structure**

If the peer review demonstrates a difference in quality outcomes, a new practice standard should be explored and implemented if the shared governance structure approves. This process of practice evolution advances new knowledge for the discipline.

Practice autonomy necessitates that multiple types of peer review processes are developed and implemented to ensure that accountability is demonstrated. Because quality and safety outcomes often require daily or hourly

**Figure 2-1.   Peer review within the nursing quality structure.**

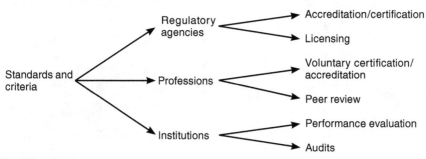

(ANA, 1988, p. 5)

monitoring, there is a need for ongoing peer review processes to alert the professional to deviations in practice.

The peer review structure also needs to address the differences between managerial and practice performance issues. If there is a practice performance issue, the peer group develops the necessary process for education, corrective action, and clinical development to ensure role actualization. Finally, the peer review structure should define credentialing and privileging for all levels and all settings of professional nursing. For practice autonomy and practitioner accountability to exist, multiple forms of peer review are needed and should be developed by the practitioners within the decisional discipline structure of shared governance.

**Table 2-1.  Systematic Literature Review on Peer Review in Nursing**

| Author | Year of Publication | Title | Topic | Location | Setting | Groups Involved | Sampling Strategy | No. of Participants |
|---|---|---|---|---|---|---|---|---|
| Altimier, L. B. | 1995 | Implementing a peer review system in neonatal ICU | Peer review program to allow nurses to formally document and provide constructive feedback to the other nurses in a NICU | America | Staff in practice | Nurses | No information | No information |
| Appling, S. E., Naumann, P. L, Berk, R. A. | 2001 | Using a faculty evaluation triad to achieve evidence-based teaching | Peer review, student evaluation and portfolio to evaluate teaching in a school of nursing | America | Staff in practice | Nurses | Not applicable | Not applicable |
| Balkizas, D., Morton, S., & Holgate, M. | 1995 | Peer accreditation of a development unit | Peer review accreditation during the formation of a nursing development unit in an LD community home | UK | Staff in practice | Nurses | Convenience | No information |

| | | | | | | | | |
|---|---|---|---|---|---|---|---|---|
| Billings, C. V. | 1998 | Professional insights: on peer feedback | Peer review to promote professional growth among nurses in a psychiatric unit | America | Staff in practice | Nurses | No information | No information |
| Breeden-Brooks, S., Olsen, P., Rieger-Kligys, S., & Mooney, L. | 1995 | Peer review: an approach to performance evaluation in a professional practice model | Peer review to increase commitment and accountability among nurses in a hospital setting | America | Staff in practice | Nurses | No information | No information |
| Buus-Frank, M. E., Conner-Bronson, J., Mullaney, D., McNamara, L. M., Laurizio, V. A., & Edwards, W. H. | 1996 | Evaluation of the neonatal nurse practitioner role: the next frontier | Peer review to evaluate the neonatal nurse practitioner role in a hospital | America | Staff in practice | Nurses | No information | No information |

*(continues)*

**Table 2-1. Systematic Literature Review on Peer Review in Nursing (Continued)**

| Author | Year of Publication | Title | Topic | Location | Setting | Groups Involved | Sampling Strategy | No. of Participants |
|---|---|---|---|---|---|---|---|---|
| Casey, J. D. | 1998 | Why do we need peer review? | Peer review to make evaluation more personalized and provide an avenue for career development and ongoing evaluation among nurses in a nursing home and a community hospital | Canada | Staff in practice | Nurses | No information | No information |
| Chang, B., Lee, J., Pearson, M., Kahn, K., Elliott, M., Rubenstein, L. | 2002 | Evaluating quality of nursing care: The gap between theory and practice | Peer review among nurses (structured implicit reviews) of in-hospital records across many hospitals | America | Staff in practice | Nurses | No information | No information |
| Cheyne, H., Niven, C., & McGinley, M. | 2003 | The PEER project: A model of peer review | Peer review to support midwifery practice and professional development in primary and secondary settings | UK | Staff in practice | Midwives | Purposive | 30 |

| | | | | | | | | | |
|---|---|---|---|---|---|---|---|---|---|
| Claveirole, A., & Mathers, M. | 2003 | Peer supervision: An experimental scheme for nurse lecturers | Peer supervision to provide education, support and quality checks for mental health nursing lecturers working in a department of nursing | UK | Staff in education | Nurses | No information | No information | No information |
| Cobb, K. L., Billings, D. M., Mays, R. M., & Canty-Mitchell, J. | 2001 | Peer review of teaching in Web-based courses in nursing | Peer review of teaching nursing on a Web-based course | America | Staff in education | Nurses | No information | No information | No information |
| Cohen, B., Berube, R., & Turrentine, B. | 1996 | A peer review program for professional nurses | Peer review to provide feedback for nurses to plan and pursue their professional growth and improve the care they provide in a university hospital | America | Staff in practice | Nurses | No information | No information | No information |

*(continues)*

**Table 2-1. Systematic Literature Review on Peer Review in Nursing (Continued)**

| Author | Year of Publication | Title | Topic | Location | Setting | Groups Involved | Sampling Strategy | No. of Participants |
|---|---|---|---|---|---|---|---|---|
| Conyers, V. | 2003 | Posters: An assessment strategy to foster learning in nursing education | Peer review of posters to stimulate learning and foster vital skills associated with information gathering, analysis and dissemination among nursing students | Australia | Students in education | Nurses | No information | No information |
| Costello, J., Pateman, B., Pusey, H., & Longshaw, K. | 2001 | Peer review of classroom teaching: An interim report | Peer review of classroom teaching in an academic department of nursing, midwifery and health visiting | UK | Staff in education | Nurses | No information | 129 |
| Dancer, S., Johnson, T., Zauner, J., & Burch, C. | 1997 | Peer evaluation. A visual picture | Peer review as part of the annual staff evaluation process for nurses working in a hospital | America | Staff in practice | Nurses | No information | No information |

| Davis, J. D. | 2002 | Comparison of faculty, peer, self and nurse assessment of obstetrics and gynaecology residents | Peer review of performance of doctors by nurses (and others) in an obstetrics and gynaecology unit | America | Staff in practice | Multi-professional | Whole population used | 16 |
|---|---|---|---|---|---|---|---|---|
| Delgado, C. & Mack, B. | 2002 | A peer-reviewed program for senior proficiencies | Peer review of student nurses clinical skills | America | Students in education | Nurses | No information | 37 |
| Engels, Y., Verheijen, N., Fleuren, M., Mokkink, H., & Grol, R. | 2003 | The effect of small peer group continuous quality improvement on the clinical practice of midwives in The Netherlands | Peer review to promote continuous quality improvement in the clinical practice of midwives in primary and secondary care | The Netherlands | Staff in practice | Midwives | No information | 255 |
| Ferguson, L. M. | 1999 | Developing students' evaluation skills | Peer review of presentations in a practice setting among students in a school of nursing | Canada | Students in practice | Nurses | No information | No information |

*(continues)*

**Table 2-1.  Systematic Literature Review on Peer Review in Nursing *(Continued)***

| Author | Year of Publication | Title | Topic | Location | Setting | Groups Involved | Sampling Strategy | No. of Participants |
|---|---|---|---|---|---|---|---|---|
| Friedman, S., & Marr, J. | 1995 | A supervisory model of professional competence: a joint service/education initiative | Peer review of clinical supervision in nursing and midwifery in a hospital | UK | Staff in practice | Nurses and midwives | No information | No information |
| Fogarty, G. B., Hornby, C., Ferguson, H. M., & Peters, L. J. | 2001 | Quality assurance in a radiation oncology unit: the chart round experience | Peer review to promote quality assurance in a radiation oncology unit (multiprofessional) | Australia | Staff in practice | Multiprofessional | No information | No information |
| Furrer, R. A. | 1996 | Implementing peer review in home health care | Peer review to provide ongoing feedback of an individual's progress at a general hospital in the department of nursing. | America | Staff in practice | Multiprofessional | Whole population used | No information |
| Gibbons, S. W., Adamo, G., Padden, D., | 2002 | Clinical evaluation in advanced | Peer review in a skills lab in a school of | America | Students in education | Nurses | No information | 27 |

| | | | | | | | | |
|---|---|---|---|---|---|---|---|---|
| Ricciardi, R., Graziano, M., Levine, E., & Hawkins, R. | | practice nursing education: using standardised patients in health assessment | nursing to evaluate clinical skills | America | Staff in practice | Multi-professional | No information | No information |
| Gillig, P. M., & Barr, A. | 1999 | A model for multidisciplinary peer review and supervision of behavioural health clinicians | Peer review to facilitate professional development in adult and child mental health and drug and alcohol service agencies including nurses | America | Staff in practice | Multi-professional | No information | No information |
| Grant, L. F., Kelley, J. H., Northington, L, & Barlow, D. | 2002 | Using TQM/CQI processes to guide development of independent and collaborative learning in two levels of baccalaureate nursing students | Peer review to promote, clinical skills, quality management and improvement among student nurses in a school of nursing | America | Students in education | Nurses | No information | No information |

*(continues)*

**Table 2-1. Systematic Literature Review on Peer Review in Nursing (Continued)**

| Author | Year of Publication | Title | Topic | Location | Setting | Groups Involved | Sampling Strategy | No. of Participants |
|---|---|---|---|---|---|---|---|---|
| Handron, D. | 1994 | Poster presentations a tool for evaluating nursing students | Peer review of students posters during a research course at an American school of nursing | America | Students in education | Nurses | No information | No information |
| Hart, G., Clinton, M., Edwards, H., Evans, K., Lunney, P., Posner, N., Tooth, B., Weir, D., & Ryan, Y. | 2000 | Accelerated professional development and peer consultation: two strategies for continuing professional education for nurses | Peer review to aid professional development among nurses working in mental health in hospital | Australia | Staff in practice | Nurses | No information | No information |
| Hostick, T. | 1995 | A shared strategy | Peer review to promote quality assurance in community MH nursing | UK | Staff in practice | Nurses | No information | No information |

| Hotko, B., & Van Dyke, D. | 1998 | Peer review strengthening leadership skills | Peer review to develop professional leadership and autonomy among nurses working in a hospital | America | Staff in practice | Nurses | No information | No information |
| Jinks, A., & Haroon-Iqbal, H. | 2004 | Peer review of clinical education 2000–2002 | Peer review of assessors during the clinical assessment of pre-reg. MH and community nurses | UK | Staff in practice | Nurses | No information | 156 |
| John-Mazza, L. | 1997 | Pearls for practice advanced practice peer review: setting new standards | Peer review of Advanced Practitioner nurses tied into job performance as well and hospital credentializing in a paediatric secondary care facility | America | Staff in practice | Nurses | Whole population used | No information |

*(continues)*

**Table 2-1.  Systematic Literature Review on Peer Review in Nursing (Continued)**

| Author | Year of Publication | Title | Topic | Location | Setting | Groups Involved | Sampling Strategy | No. of Participants |
|---|---|---|---|---|---|---|---|---|
| Larson, J. L., & Herrick, C. | 1996 | Peer review in a shared governance model | Peer review to re-evaluate personal performance, to plan for individual goals, foster accountability, provide empowerment to those who use it and to show trends of performance in the unit as a whole among nurses in a hospital | America | Staff in practice | Nurses | Whole population used | No information |
| Ludwick, R., Cline Diekman, B., Herdtner, S., Dugan, M., & Roche, M. | 1998 | Documenting the scholarship of clinical teaching through peer review | Peer review of clinical skills teachers is an academic department of nursing | America | Staff in education | Nurses | No information | No information |

| Malby, R., & Manning, S. | 1998 | Promoting change through peer review | Peer review to provide personal development and support for nurse leaders across a whole Trusts | UK | Staff in practice | Nurses | No information | No information | No information |
|---|---|---|---|---|---|---|---|---|---|
| Malkin, K. F. | 1994 | A standard for professional development: the use of self and peerreview; learning contracts and reflection in clinical practice | Peer review to promote individual professional accountability on a ward in nursing | UK | Staff in practice | Nurses | No information | No information | No information |
| Martsolf, D. S., Dieckman, B. C., & Heiss, M. A. | 1998 | Cultural factors related to the peer review of teaching | Peer review of teaching across several university departments including nursing | America | Staff in practice | Nurses | No information | No information | 24 |

*(continues)*

**Table 2-1.   Systematic Literature Review on Peer Review in Nursing *(Continued)***

| Author | Year of Publication | Title | Topic | Location | Setting | Groups Involved | Sampling Strategy | No. of Participants |
|--------|---------------------|-------|-------|----------|---------|-----------------|-------------------|---------------------|
| Mathews, D. E. | 2000 | Developing a perioperative peer performance appraisal system | Peer review program to allow nurses to evaluate their peers' performance of activities important to px or department outcomes in a surgical unit | America | Staff in practice | Nurses | No information | No information |
| McAllister, M., & Osborne, Y. | 1997 | Peer review a strategy to enhance cooperative student learning | Peer review to enhance cooperative learning in MH undergraduate nursing students in a school of nursing | Australia | Students in education | Nurses | No information | No information |
| McDermott, J., Buffington, S. T., Prenggono, D, & Achadi, E. | 2001 | Two models of in-service training to improve midwifery skills: how well do they work? | Peer review as part of competency-based skill training and continuing education among midwives working in secondary care | Indonesia | Staff in practice | Midwives | No information | No information |

| | | | | | | | | |
|---|---|---|---|---|---|---|---|---|
| Micheli, A. J., & Modest, S. | 1995 | Peer review | Peer review program for nurses to evaluate performance at a children's hospital | America | Staff in practice | Nurses | No information | No information |
| Mitchell, M, Hunt, C, Johnson, J, Ovitt, B, & Lemon, D. | 1995 | Enhancing peer review with communication skill building | Peer review to provide feedback to staff in order to meet personal, professional, departmental or hospital expectations among nurses | America | Staff in practice | Nurses | No information | No information |
| Parks, J., & Lindstrom, C. W. | 1995 | Taking the fear out of peer review | Peer review to promote professional development, fosters a group philosophy and provides a forum for recognition among psychiatric nurses | America | Staff in practice | Nurses | No information | No information |

*(continues)*

**Table 2-1.  Systematic Literature Review on Peer Review in Nursing (Continued)**

| Author | Year of Publication | Title | Topic | Location | Setting | Groups Involved | Sampling Strategy | No. of Participants |
|---|---|---|---|---|---|---|---|---|
| Pedersen, A., Crabtree, T., & Ortiz-Tomei, T. | 2004 | Implementation of the peer review council | Peer review (multiprofessional) to help develop unit cultures of professionalism, involvement and excellence, and overcome problems such as late evaluations and discipline specific reviews in hospital | America | Staff in practice | Nurses | Convenience | No information |
| Ribbons, B., & Vance, S. | 2001 | Using e-mail to facilitate nursing scholarship | Peer review via e-mail to promote 1st year undergraduate nursing students' understanding of scholarship in a school of nursing | Australia | Students in education | Nurses | No information | No information |
| Richardson, C., & Schmeiser, D. N. | 2001 | Staff colleagues evaluate clinical faculty | Peer review of teaching in a school of nursing | America | Staff in education | Nurses | No information | No information |

| | | | | | | | | |
|---|---|---|---|---|---|---|---|---|
| Roper, K. A., & Russell, G. | 1997 | The effect of peer review on professionalism, autonomy and accountability | Peer review program for nurses intended to improve and foster professionalism, accountability and px satisfaction in an in-px haematology/oncology unit. Planning only | America | Staff in practice | Nurses | No information | No information |
| Sedlak, C. A., & O'Bryan Doheny, M. | 1998 | Peer review through clinical rounds a collaborative critical thinking strategy | Peer review through student-led clinical rounds in an acute care setting to promote student's critical thinking in communicating assessment data and identifying client strengths and problems. | America | Students in practice | Nurses | No information | 19 |

*(continues)*

**Table 2-1.  Systematic Literature Review on Peer Review in Nursing *(Continued)***

| Author | Year of Publication | Title | Topic | Location | Setting | Groups Involved | Sampling Strategy | No. of Participants |
|---|---|---|---|---|---|---|---|---|
| Sheahan, S. L., Simpson, C., & Rayens, M. K. | 2001 | Nurse practitioner peer review: process and evaluation | Peer review program to improve client outcomes and promote optimum practice standards for Nurse Practitioners in a hospital | America | Staff in practice | Nurses | No information | 15 |
| Smith, M. A., Atherly, A. J., Kane, R. L., & Pacala, J. T. | 1997 | Peer review of the quality of care reliability and sources of variability for outcome and process assessments | Peer review to compare interrater reliability of review of charts by disciplines including nurses in acute and long-term care for frail older adults | America | Staff in practice | Multiprofessional | No information | No information |
| Stein, E. | 1996 | Peer review in a New York chapter of the ACNM 1987–1994 | Peer review of midwifery care by evaluating standards, processes and outcomes in all | America | Staff in practice | Midwives | Convenience | No information |

| Vezina, M., Chiang, J., Laufer, K., Garabedian, C., Padre, H., & Sanders, N. | 1996 | Competency-based orientation for clinical nurse educators | Peer review to successfully assimilate new educators into the roles of clinical expert and teacher among nurses in an American hospital ... institutions in one geographical area | America | Staff in practice | Nurses | No information | No information |
|---|---|---|---|---|---|---|---|---|
| Willson, L., Fawcett, T. N., & Whyte, D. A. | 2001 | An evaluation of a clinical supervision programme | Peer review to provide formalised support linked with practice review and professional development that aimed to enhance the delivery of px care among community nurses | UK | Staff in practice | Nurses | No information | No information |

Source: "Peer Review in Nursing and Midwifery: A Literature Review," by A. Rout and P. Roberts, 2006, *Journal of Clinical Nursing, 17*, 4, pp. 433–440. Copyright 2007 by Blackwell Publishing Ltd. Reprinted with permission.

## REFERENCES

American Nurses Association. (1976). *One strong voice: The story of American Nurses Association.* Kansas City, MO: Author.

American Nurses Association. (1988). *Peer review in nursing practice.* Kansas City, MO: Author.

American Nurses Association. (2003). *Nursing's social policy statement* (2nd ed.). Washington, DC: Author.

Brooks, S., Olsen P., Rieger-Kligys, S., & Mooney, L. (1995). Peer review: An approach to performance evaluation in professional practice model. *Critical Care Nursing Quarterly, 18*(3), 36–47.

Cheyne, H., Niven, C., & McGinley, M. (2003). The PEER project: A model of peer review. *British Journal of Midwifery, 11*(4), 227–232.

Cohen, B., Berube, R., & Turrentine, B. (1996, Jan/Feb). A peer review program for professional nurses. *Journal of Nursing Staff Development, 12*(1), 13–18.

Dossey, B. M., Selanders, L. C., Beck, D. M., & Attewell, A. (2005). *Florence Nightingale today: Healing, leadership, global action.* Silver Spring, MD: American Nurses Association.

Greenwood, E. (1957). Attributes of a profession. *Social Work, 2*(5), 44–45.

Larson, J. & Herrick, C. (1996). Peer review in a shared governance model. *Journal of Peri-Anesthesia Nursing, 11*(5), 317–323.

Pedersen, A. (2004, June). Implementation of the peer review council. *MedSurg Nursing.* Available at: http://findarticles.com/p/articles/mi_m0FSS/is_3_13/ai_n17207180/?tag=content;col1. Accessed January 9, 2010.

Porter-O'Grady, T. & Finnigan, S. (1984). *Shared governance for nursing a creative approach to professional accountability.* Rockville, MD: Aspen Systems Corp.

Rout, A., & Roberts, P. (2007). Peer review in nursing and midwifery: A literature review. *Journal of Clinical Nursing, 17,* 4, 427–442. doi: 10.1111/j.1365-2702.2007.01934.x

Sedlak, C., & Doheny, M. (1998). Peer review through clinical rounds: A collaborative critical thinking strategy. *Nurse Educator, 23*(5), 42–45.

Wojcik, J. (2009). Hospitals fall short on safety, quality: Leapfrog. Available at: http://www.businessinsurance.com/cgi-bin/printStory.pl?news_id=15959. Accessed April 29, 2009.

# CHAPTER 3

# A Conceptual Model for Professional Peer Review

*Man's mind, stretched to a new idea,*
*never goes back to its original dimensions.*

—OLIVER WENDELL HOLMES

## ELEMENTS OF THE MODEL

The concept of peer review is grounded in the principles of professionalism. The ultimate outcome of professionalism is held in the public trust as each professional agrees to advocate on the public's behalf. In doing so, professionals hold themselves accountable to the standards of the profession and the standards and care of their practice. The public puts their trust in the profession and agrees that it must have the authority to act autonomously and be fearless if they recognize a breech of ethics. The promise of the nursing discipline as a collective in any organized setting is to ensure that the principles of autonomous practice are in balance with the current standards and that the practice is defined by the evidence of all disciplines that contribute any new research knowledge to the delivery of patient care.

Autonomous nursing practice must also provide a frame of reference for the peer review process. The peer review process should focus on how the individual's practice performance matches the standards developed by the collective. In an organized setting of practice with multiple practitioners, it is the responsibility of the collective to organize a structure and process to ensure that peer review is conducted. Peer review processes within a framework of a nursing quality assurance plan ensure that safety and quality care are provided. These processes also become a reference point for understanding the patterns of growth and development of the practitioner and the development of new standards determined by the practice outcomes. The individual practitioner and the performance standards of the discipline define the relationship to the client or patient served.

47

**Conceptual Model of Peer Review**

In describing the concept of peer review in an organized setting where one discipline of nursing coexists with multiple other practitioners, the work is complex and multivariate. The role of each practitioner must be defined and understood by all collective groups if the system is to thrive. A conceptual model is a way of describing a framework to connect all roles and all elements of a dynamic, fluid, and organizational relationship-based system. A conceptual peer review model is illustrated in Figure 3-1.

The theoretical framework for this model is a synthesis of elements and evidence-based practice processes described in the research literature. A systems approach is used to showcase the complexity and interconnectedness of all of the parts. The model is applicable to all disciplines attempting to structure a peer review process. Utilizing Ford's (1992) motivational systems theory approach to behavior change or achievement, one can balance the variables of motivation, acquisition of skill, and a responsive environment with the

**Figure 3-1.   Conceptual model of peer review.**

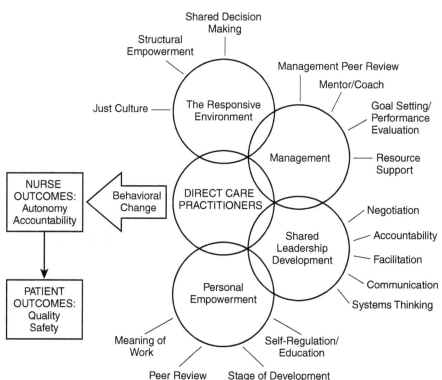

concept of outcomes from peer review. For the professional, the outcomes are autonomy and accountability. For the patient, the outcomes are quality and safety of care.

## Theoretical Aspects of the Model

Motivation, as a concept, was informed by the leadership/goal/feedback theory as described by Yulk and Latham (1978). The responsive environment was informed by Kanter's (1979) theory of management. Skill acquisition and behavior was informed by Bandura's (1977) self-efficacy theory. Other researchers, such as Manojlovich (2005), have framed a reference of motivation to self-efficacy theory and nursing practice autonomy. Self-efficacy refers to a belief in one's capabilities to organize and mobilize the motivation and cognitive resources, and execute the courses of action needed to produce a given result (Bandura). To identify the appropriate course of action and definitively function as professionals, nurses must have an understanding of and control over the entire spectrum of activities associated with nursing an organized setting and the belief in their ability to do so. Without the autonomy to make decisions about practice, and therefore frame a process around peer review, nurses may not be able to work effectively or collectively in a manner consistent with professional standards.

## Quality and Safety Outcomes

A major assumption of the model is that staff nurses' professional practice autonomy and decision making are related to the quality and safety outcomes of the patients under their care. Maas and Jacox's (1977) research supports this assertion and concluded a clear relationship exists between the quality of the service direct care nurses provide and the extent to which they perceive themselves able to function autonomously in decisions regarding their care. Aiken, Smith, and Lake's (1994) and Aiken, Sochalski, and Lake's (1997) studies show nurses affect patient outcomes by their direct actions and their influence over the action of others. Their studies suggested that patients were favorably affected when models of management resulted in staff nurses having greater autonomy at the point of care. A recent report from researchers at Brigham and Women's hospital (Rothschild, 2006) found that not only were nurses accountable for their own practice but they were also seen as responsible for intercepting the serious errors in critically ill patients. Nurses in this study recovered 42% of the medical errors that potentially would have harmed the patient if not questioned by the nurse. This phenomenon of rescuing the patient from harm is not new to the profession of nursing but, as demonstrated in this case, does not happen with regularity of a systems approach. Many would conclude that a process of peer review that occurs not intermittently, but as an on going process built into the daily practice of review of care would seem a necessary component to always ensure that "no failure to rescue" occurs and that patients are kept safe from harm. These researchers concluded that nurses need to understand how important their role is in patient care by being more knowledgeable and more communicative with others when they suspect problems that can affect patient outcomes. The researchers go on to hypothesize why nurses feel they sometimes cannot communicate with others about these potential problems. Another example of this barrier to communication is evidenced in the 2005 study titled *Silence Kills* (Vital Smarts, 2005). In this clinical study of 1700 RNs, MDs, clinical care staff, and administrators, the researchers found that less than 10% of respondents addressed poor behavior in colleagues. Poor behaviors included trouble following direction, poor clinical judgment, and taking dangerous short cuts that affected patient safety and care. The answer to resolving these issues for professionals could lie in the next element of this conceptual model, the responsive environment. Clearly, there is a need for a cultural change lead by transformational leadership and structural empowerment.

## The Responsive Environment: Structural Empowerment

In a report for the Brookings Institution, Levine and D'Andrea (Manning & Curtis, 2003) reviewed all the major studies of empowerment in the work place. Their findings are summed up in a few words: Employee participation has a positive impact on business success. Laschinger and Shamian (1994) and Laschinger, Sabiston, and Kutszcher (1997) found that direct care nurses felt more empowered in their work settings when their managers encouraged autonomy, facilitative decision making, and expressed confidence in employee competence. Kanter (1979) argues that employees' behaviors are a reaction to the situation in which they find themselves. In the discussion of structural empowerment, Kanter believes that the growth of empowerment is related to employees' access to information and resources, to receiving support, and to having the opportunity to learn and grow. According to Kanter, the mandate for management is to create conditions of work effectiveness by ensuring that all employees have access to information, support, and resources necessary to do their work. When employees have these elements of structural empowerment, it increases feelings of autonomy, higher levels of self-efficacy and self-confidence, and greater commitment to the organization.

## The Responsive Environment: The Manager's Role

The manager's role in resource allocation is to ensure that the professionals have the necessary resources and supplies to carry out the work of the discipline. This means that managers must support the structural design of shared governance and resource it appropriately if the work of self-regulation is to be successful.

Supporting the staff by providing the necessary data and information to the unit councils helps the staff to make better decisions. Management creates and supports a just culture by providing all the data on clinical outcomes and the education necessary to help the staff see the areas of improvement needed.

It would be hard for a unit-based council to be held accountable to improving clinical outcomes of care if the members of the council never saw or were coached to look for the data necessary to evaluate the current state of care. In the unit-based and organization-wide councils, the building and developing of a peer review model that will improve outcomes, whether that means a system change or a personal practitioner improvement plan, is the council's accountability. The manager's role is to support, plan, and provide the resources for protected time. This protected time to participate in council work is often budgeted by finance as nonproductive time and removed from the budget during cost reduction periods. Managers need to partner with finance to relabel and redefine protective time as productive. Another important management function is to share data on financial and clinical outcomes with the staff in the shared governance structure. This data has traditionally been the purview of management and not transparent to the staff. The staff structures of practice and professional peer review can be held accountable to the cost and quality improvements in clinical care and patient satisfaction if they have the data and are involved in the decisions to improve outcomes. This is how management supports structural empowerment and creates the responsive environment.

### The Manager's Role in Coaching and Mentoring

Haag-Heitman (2008) found in her research that development of expert practice in direct care nurses was influenced by the role of the very first frontline supervisor. Study participants commented that as novice nurses, they felt supported by managers who challenged the status quo and role modeled the communication necessary to affect change. The manager's role model created the environment for these developing nurses to also become strong patient advocates, which helped them challenge the other members of the healthcare team. When managers create environments that are conducive to good communication, like giving and receiving feedback and conflict management, staff feel encouraged and supported to do the same. Participants also described that manager's modeled skilled communication, collaboration, and patient advocacy.

### The Manager's Role in Reward and Recognition

Applied behavioral scientists have shown that using the principles of goal setting, feedback on performance, and positive reinforcement has been shown to have a positive impact on employee performance and engagement (Manning & Curtis, 2003). Managers who recognize and reward all aspects of the peer review process at all levels and settings of nursing practice will see increased staff participation in the design and implementation of new innovations in peer review. Unit goals will be accomplished by these high performing teams because staff will take ownership for the process of improving patient care outcomes. Transformational leaders set the milieu of this responsive environment through rewarding and recognizing the early adopters and innovators of the process. Those who take a risk at peer review are seen by others as the champions for patient care change and are recognized by leadership in public forums. The manager creates the responsive environment that is supportive of the implementation of the staff designed peer review process. The manager's role is also instructive, by role modeling the behavior of peer review within the manager-designed peer review process. When the staff sees this role modeling by managers, they begin to trust that peer review is not a punitive system, but is an equity-based system applicable to all clinicians.

### Shared Decision Making: Staff and Manager's Roles

Professional nurses, like colleagues in all disciplines, should be active participants in most unit and organizational operational decisions. Operations by definition would seem to include all staff types in all roles on the unit that is charged with the implementation process. It is what the concept of participatory management is built upon. Often, however, in participatory management, the staff is involved only as much as the managers need them to operationally implement the manager's decision. It is common in a complex healthcare system that this decision is often seen by staff as not being implemented. It is not uncommon to find in complex healthcare systems that a manager's decisions are often viewed by the staff as not acceptable because they cannot be implemented in the way they were designed. The manager simply does not have the knowledge necessary to make clinical decisions that will impact the patients under the clinician's care. This is why managers who move to models of shared decision making are successful.

In shared decision making processes, outcomes of implementation are more successful because staff own their part in the actual decision to implement. The time to get to the actual decision might take a little longer in the processing part of the equation, but the implementation timeline more than makes up for this loss. Implementation not only goes faster, but there is also a commitment on the part of staff to its sustainability, rather than to rule compliance, which ultimately diminishes over time. An old adage describes this process well: "The person in the boat with you never bores a hole in it."

### Shared Decision Making Case Study

This case study illustrates the concepts of shared decision-in-action, moving away from traditional management roles of directing and controlling. It focuses on the redesign and expansion of an Emergency Department.

Traditionally, the Emergency Department manager sits on the design committee for creating a large square foot expansion of the a unit. In shared decision making, the manager engages the already established unit-based council members to partner in the decision and attend the design meetings. Traditionally, the manager would simply post the architectural plans for design of the new unit and ask for comments. In shared decision making, the team is involved in the planning process and in the actual decision making for creating the new operational environment. In this process of design decision making, those involved would have taken ownership of their decisions and returned to the unit level staff for their ideas. In the traditional model, the new unit might look great to the manager who designed it, but staff might feel stressed as they try to care for patients in the new environment. Many staff might feel alienated and voice the discontent at not having the opportunity to be involved in the design of the unit. In shared decision making, the new design plan and a new care delivery system is developed. The design and plan for improvement of operations is communicated, and conflicts resolved before the unit is opened, making the move less stressful. When staff take ownership for their practice and the practice environment, they are more engaged in process improvement and more satisfied with the work environment.

## Manager's Role in Shared Decision Making

In shared decision making, managers must be knowledgeable about the balance between operational and practice decisions. When the process of shared decision making occurs, successful outcomes are produced. When managers are clear as to the role of the staff in defining the professional discipline's work of self-regulation, then staff feel empowered to make decisions. The professional roles of manager and of staff are seen as separate but integrated into the work of the unit's practice and operational structure as illustrated in Figure 3-2.

### *The Manager's Role in Goal Setting and Performance Evaluation*

In both laboratory and field studies, 90% of the research conducted supported a notion of participation by employees in the goal setting process along with the use of prior performance. This leads to specific and challenging goals, which, in turn, leads to higher performance. Goals and feedback affected performance by driving attention, mobilizing effort, increasing persistence, and motivating strategy development (Locke, Shaw, Saari & Latham, 1981). Chances for success are strengthened as one organizes, designs, or modifies tasks, activities, and experiences so he or she can afford the attainment of as many different goals as possible. Goals must constantly meet optimal challenges for the individual. In the context of the workplace, the goal setting process should be the role of management with the participation of the individual for whom the goals are written. The manager's role is to ensure that, through the performance evaluation and goal setting process,

**Figure 3-2.   Staff and manager's roles in shared leadership.**

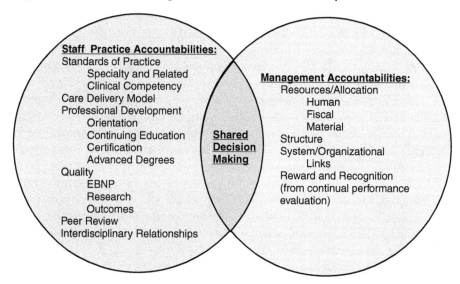

the demands of the person's professional goals are in concert with the goals of the organization and the strategic plan for the discipline. The manager's role is to ensure congruence between goals and accomplishments and the reward and recognition strategies, both intrinsic and extrinsic. This process typically occurs between the manager and staff at the time of the annual performance review. For example, the manager and staff during the goal setting timeframe would understand that the goal of the discipline and the goal of the organization might be to achieve magnet recognition status. In order to do so, the discipline must promote and record all those nurses who are certified in their clinical and administrative specialty. The unit goal for the manager- and unit-based council might be to increase certification rates to benchmark with like Magnet (R) hospital units. When coaching the staff, the manager might indicate that certification is a unit goal and therefore should be a goal for all eligible staff. During the time of goal setting with each staff member, a goal is written related to certification where appropriate for each staff member as an opportunity for the next year's professional organizational work. During the performance evaluation process the following year, the staff is rewarded for having achieved the goal.

### Role of Feedback

An additional key strategy to goal setting is the use of feedback for the purposes of growth and development. Yulk and Latham (1978) demonstrated that feedback alone was insufficient to improve performance, but feedback along with goal setting did increase performance and results. In both laboratory and field studies, 90% indicated that specific and challenging goals lead to a higher performance than did easy goals (George, 1999a). It takes management skills to coach and mentor this type of goal-setting process. Performance evaluations should be a measure of recognition and reward for accomplishing challenging goal assignments.

### Goal Setting in Peer Review

Clinical peer review between practitioners of like rank should be another focus for goal setting. The feedback about one's clinical performance from peers should guide the practitioner to develop new goals related to practice expectations and outcomes. For example, if the discipline frames an annual feedback tool for staff from others of similar rank in the same unit, then the purpose of this feedback is supported by management but not owned by management. Staff is supported to seek out this feedback either verbally or in written format by asking the other staff on the unit for direct, open, and honest feedback. The key elements of this feedback are that this not be anonymous and that each person in the unit must participate in some way during the process. One easy way to accomplish an equally participative process is to randomly assign all staff to do the peer review based on similar characteristics, such as shifts worked or career ladder attainment. The format of the peer review should be based on practice performance, not the employee values of the organization. Those values are better suited for a round of 360 feedbacks, which are not considered a form of peer review because typically it is not done with staff of peers. The peer review feedback should go directly and confidentially back to the person being reviewed. That staff person has an opportunity to seek out a coach to help interpret the feedback and to assist him or her in establishing an achievable goal that he or she, in turn, can bring to his or her goal setting session with his or her manager. Using feedback can be a powerful tool for behavioral change once integrated to the process of establishing goals and performance evaluation.

### The Manager's Peer Review

Peer review for managers ensures that equity as a principle of shared governance is maintained within the system of managers. In this model, all managers see themselves as part of the discipline of nursing regardless of reporting relationship to the chief nursing officer or any other leader. As a part of the whole system, each manager participates in the discipline goal setting process as a way of establishing like goals for system and like performance objectives for the person. For example, the professional development council may say that all professional nursing staff will have a personal professional development plan. This would mean the management council adopts a strategy to ensure that this happens and asks each nursing manager to see to it that each professional staff member has a professional development plan. Each manager helps the staff establish a unique goal associated with that plan. If one manager does not do this task as assigned, then there is no equity in the system. Managers use peer review to ensure that the goal is accomplished.

### Personal Empowerment

Incorporated into the concept of self-regulation is the individual's willingness to make the personal engagement necessary to do the work. Shared visions create a sense of ownership and professional connectedness to the discipline and/or to the organization depending on the practice setting. Spreitzer (1996) defines this concept as psychological empowerment. It contains the concepts of autonomy and self-efficacy, both outcomes of a responsive environment.

Psychological empowerment occurs in four personal constructs: meaning of the work, competence to do the work, self-determination, and impact of the outcomes on the work. These four constructs define an active orientation to the role and a framework for motivation to perform peer review. Understanding the relationship of this research to the tenets of the professional practice is key to the successful alignment of both the professional's work and also personal empowerment.

All nurses play a critical role in the legitimization of the professional practice environment. Each professional requires continuous learning, engagement in the collective decision making structure, a personal commitment to peer review, and an established ability to develop a practice model based on beliefs and attitudes of the discipline. These elements of participation should be discussed with the professional before the hiring process takes place. Not unlike the medical staff, nursing as a professional discipline should create its own set of rules and regulations related to professional engagement. Professional nurses should understand they are joining the discipline of nursing within an organizational context. By being granted the privilege of joining this professional association, they must first understand that participation in the work of governance is not optional. There are two forms of participation, active and passive. The level of participation is determined by the discipline in terms of its bylaws.

The medical staff model has sustained a significant level of power and autonomy. Each medical staff model defines expectations for participation in the governance model for membership in the organization. Through this medical staff model, a process of peer review for assessing the level of professional participation occurs. The model of recredentialing and privileging by the profession for the professional is the key to sustainability of the profession and its professional relationship with the organization.

This is not the work of management but the work of the professional practicing in the discipline. Peers should therefore be involved in the interview of new hires, and the granting of privileges to practice as defined by the shared governance bylaws. The rules of employee–employer engagement are also important and must be discussed during the same interviewing process by the manager.

Personal empowerment occurs as the individual engages in the meaning of the work. Competence to do the work is established using the credentialing process of peer review. Self-determination occurs in the active participation of governance and the achievement of work outcomes.

### Shared Leadership Development

It is important that all practitioners are grounded in the principles of shared leadership education (George *et al.*, 2002). Training staff on the shared leadership constructs of systems thinking, facilitation skills, accountability, and negotiation confirmed that leadership and professional autonomy behaviors can be significantly increased (George, 1999b). It is important to provide a shared leadership training program to support successful leadership for peer review.

Leaders in formal roles must also be familiar with the components of shared leadership training. As managers engage in the peer review of each other, they are grounded in these transformational behaviors. A fuller description of shared leadership training is presented in Chapter 6.

### Integrating the Conceptual Model

Peer review in nursing as a professional construct has been promoted by the American Nurses Association since the early 1970s. The literature, however, is mostly void of any actual work done in this area. This conceptual framework based on system motivational theory and the concepts of self-efficacy and personal empowerment is a model from which new designs of peer review may evolve. All elements of the model are interrelated and should not be undertaken individually. For example, attempting to do a shared leadership training program for direct care nurses where they would then enter back into a nonresponsive environment would be just as unsuccessful as building a shared governance structure of peer review that is not properly resourced or does not provide accurate data to assess competence. The key to success in these processes of peer review is that all elements of the conceptual framework are aligned to the structure and processes of the organization and are fully implemented in all areas of practice and at all levels of the nursing hierarchy. Peer review guidelines must be written and the structure must be implemented within the individual units and the system as a whole. In addition, the elements of the peer review process must be done by the members of a peer group. One of the most significant and visible decisions that must be entertained is how to separate the concepts of peer review from the annual performance evaluation done under the management domain. Separating clinical advancement and peer review from a yearly performance evaluation done by management allows for the direct care practitioner to focus daily feedback on clinical excellence. This peer feedback process is modeled in the shared leadership and communication training program and must be fostered by management in the responsive environment. Relationships between peers are based on peer trust and mutual respect. A climate of trust builds among all members of the team as the personal and unit goals are achieved and the outcomes for improved quality and safety are demonstrated.

Before improvements in quality and safety can occur, the structure for peer review must be built and aligned to the self-regulation structures of the organization. The next chapter details the integration of peer review into a professional practice environment structured through shared governance.

## REFERENCES

Aiken, L. H., Smith, H. L., & Lake, E. T. (1994). Lower Medicare mortality among a set of hospitals known for good nursing care. *Medical Care, 32*(8), 771–787.

Aiken, L. H., Sochalski, J., & Lake, E. T. (1997). Studying outcomes of organizational change in health services. *Medical Care, 35*(11), NS6–NS18.

Bandura, A. (1977). Self-efficacy: Toward a unifying theory of behavioral change. *Psychological Review, 84*(2), 191–215.

Ford, M. (1992). *Motivating humans: Goals, emotions, and personal agency beliefs.* Thousand Oaks, CA: Sage.

George, V. (1999a). *An organizational case study in shared leadership* (Unpublished doctoral dissertation). Marquette University College of Nursing, Milwaukee, WI.

George, V. (1999b). The role of the chief nurse executive in fostering excellence in the professional practice environment. In B. Haag-Heitman (Ed.), *Clinical practice development using novice to expert theory* (pp. 229–239). Gaithersburg, MD: Aspen.

George, V., Burke, L., Rodgers, B., Duthie, N., Hoffman, M.L., Koceja, V., *et al.* (2002). Developing staff nurse shared leadership behavior in professional practice. *Nursing Administrative Quarterly, 26*(3), 44–59.

Haag-Heitman, B. (2008). The development of expert performance in nursing. *Journal for Nurses in Staff Development, 24*(5), 203–211.

Kanter, R. M. (1979). *Men and women of the corporation.* New York: Basic Books.

Laschinger, H. K., Sabiston, J. A., & Kutszcher, L. (1997). Empowerment and staff nurse decision involvement in nursing work environment: Testing Kanter's theory of structural power in organizations. *Research in Nursing and Health, 20*(4), 341–352.

Laschinger, H. K., & Shamian, J. (1994). Staff nurses' and nurse managers' perceptions of job-related empowerment and managerial self-efficacy. *Journal of Nursing Administration, 24*(10), 38–47.

Locke, E., Shaw, K., Saari, L., & Latham, G. (1981). Goal setting and task performance. *Psychological Bulletin, 90*(1), 125–152.

Maas, M., & Jacox, A. (1977). *Guideline for nurse autonomy/patient welfare.* New York, NY: Appleton-Century-Crofts.

Manning, G., & Curtis, K. (2003). *The art of leadership.* Boston: McGraw-Hill.

Manojlovich, M. (2005). Promoting nurses' self-efficacy: A leadership strategy to improve practice. *Journal of Nursing Administration, 35*(5), 271–278.

Rothschild, J. M. (2006). Recovery from medical errors: The critical care nursing safety net. *The Joint Commission Journal on Quality and Patient Safety, 32*(2), 63–72.

Spreitzer, G. (1996). Social structural characteristics of psychological empowerment. *Academy of Management Journal, 39*(2), 483–504.

VitalSmarts. (2006). *Silence kills: The seven crucial conversations for healthcare.* Available at: www.silencekills.com. Accessed February 14, 2010.

Yulk, G., & Latham, G. (1978). Interrelationship among employee participation, individual differences, goal difficulty, goal acceptances, goal instrumentality, and performance. *Personnel Psychology, 31*, 305–307.

# CHAPTER 4

# Using Shared Governance Structures for Peer Review Integration

*Do not go where the path may lead, go instead where there is no path and leave a trail.*

—Ralph Waldo Emerson

The authors of the American Nurses' Association (ANA) peer review guidelines recognized that organizational performance is influenced by structural factors and that successful implementation of peer review requires an organized effort and systematic approach. This chapter describes how to organize the effort of integrating peer review in an organization's shared governance structure. Dr. Donabedian's (1988) quality and performance improvement model emphasizes that the environment or structure in which health care is provided can constrain performance improvement processes. In nursing, shared governance is the time-tested structure that promotes self-regulation and the achievement of professional outcomes. Therefore, shared governance is endorsed as the structure for peer review. This chapter presents structural principles, guidelines, models, accountabilities, and recommendations for shared governance models to promote peer review integration.

## FOUNDATIONAL PROGRAM GUIDELINES

The program guidelines section for peer review from the ANA provides a foundation for the guiding principles to operationalize peer review programs:

> Peer review as an organized program requires written, standardized operation procedures developed and adopted by the nurses to be reviewed and by appropriate administrative bodies. The document should state (a) the intent of the peer review program in a particular setting, (b) the way the finding of peer review will be used, (c) the method of selecting reviewers, (d) the responsibilities of nurse reviewers and of management for the peer review program, and (e) the time frame for periodic reviews or conditions under which special reviews may be conducted. In settings where self-governance or shared governance is practiced, nursing bylaws should describe the structure and functions of the peer review program.

61

The peer review program must provide for confidentiality with regard to patient care records and must honor the rights of the nurses being reviewed, the reviewers, the clients, the nurse administrators, and other professionals who share responsibility for patient care.

The quality, quantity, and cost of the peer review program itself require monitoring. The operating procedures should provide for maintenance of records of the peer review process and programs to permit evaluation of their efficiency and effectiveness in relation to their cost.

Since essentially the same steps are used in peer review as in other kinds of nursing practice evaluation, the seven steps in the ANA model of quality assurance in nursing are used here to organize the elements of the peer review program.

1. Identify values. The peer group should reach consensus on which values underlying its area of practice are relevant to peer review in the specific situation. These values should be consistent with the philosophy of the nursing service department of the agency. The values should reflect the Code for Nurses, standards of practice, and other documents of the nursing profession.
2. Identify standards and criteria. Specific structure, process, and outcome standards relevant to the setting should be identified. Related measurable criteria should then be elaborated as a basis for judging nursing practice decisions and the quality of care resulting from the decision process. It is important for the whole group of peers, at least through representatives, to be involved in developing and adopting the standards and criteria that will be used to judge their practice.
3. Secure measurements. The methods for securing the descriptive or quantified data necessary for determining the degree to which standards of practice and related criteria have been met should be established before their use in the peer review process. The peer group or designated representatives should participate in the selection of data collection methods and the time frame for their use. Methods may vary from record audits to examination of reimbursement claims referred for review of nursing care.
4. Make interpretations. The nurse reviewers analyze the data in light of the agreed-on standards and criteria and make judgments about strengths, deficits, or other problems in quality. Further, they analyze decision points to determine that appropriate nursing care decisions were made in a timely fashion. The nursing care delivered as a result of the nursing decisions is further evaluated for its necessity, efficiency, and effectiveness, particularly when the review is associated with third-party reimbursement.
5. Identify courses of action. The nurse reviewers identify suitable courses of action to reward strengths, correct deficits, solve problems, and prevent later problems whenever possible.
6. Choose actions. According to the operating procedures previously defined, the nurse reviewers choose or recommend selected courses of action.

If the action is to recommend, it should be directed to the most appropriate group for action. Provisions should be made for appealing the reviewers' decisions.

7. Take action. If empowered to do so, the nurse reviewers take the action chosen. Otherwise, they should obtain reports of follow-up on the actions recommended to others. The both cases, the results of recommended actions should be evaluated by peer review groups. (ANA, 1988, pp. 7–9)

## BUILDING PEER REVIEW STRUCTURES AND PROCESSES

Kanter's (1979) research on empowerment in the workplace found that organizational structure is an important correlate of behavior in organizations. In nursing, shared governance provides the empowerment structure for achieving meaningful professional behaviors and outcomes. When staff and management make decisions using the shared governance principles of partnership, equity, ownership, and accountability, the process of authentic shared decision making occurs. The outcome of this shared decision making process is shared leadership. Figure 4-1 illustrates these relationships in a self-regulation organizational framework.

**Figure 4-1.   The model of self-regulation.**

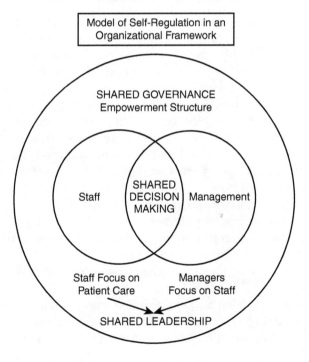

If your organization does not have a shared governance structure, this is where you must begin. If your organization already has shared governance, you need to examine your structure to ensure that you have fully integrated and implemented all forms of peer review management under a self-regulation model. Remember, practice autonomy necessitates that multiple types of peer review processes are developed and implemented to assure that accountability for this autonomy is demonstrated. This includes: (1) role actualization, using the beginner-to-expert model; (2) practice advancement, including the credentialing and privileging processes for nurses at all levels (including management), and (3) quality and safety processes, to alert professionals to deviations in practice standards and to advance the discipline by giving feedback on quality and safety to learning to each individual practitioner and to the discipline as a whole. Shared governance is the structure needed to formally review the professional practice quality and safety outcomes at both the organization and unit-based levels. Through this process, quality and safety become key agenda items at each shared governance council meeting. The shared governance membership designs the steps necessary to improve outcomes using the peer review process.

## ORGANIZING THE EFFORTS

### Role of Management—Creating the Shared Vision

A shared vision for health care parallels the changes in industry in which one must account for not only the changing demographics of the workforce (Boyett & Conn, 1991), but also the quality-based consumer-directed movement. This shared vision requires leaders and followers to put a structure in place that fosters shared decision making. Contemporary management practice indicates that the most successful businesses are those that empower the staff at the point of service to act with freedom and responsibility. In order to act with freedom and responsibility, the staff needs to engage in the strategic prioritization and decisions that affect the future of that business. In health care, patients are also involved in the decisions that impact their care. Consumers expect a healthcare partner that will engage them in a discussion about options and choice. Therefore, building a shared vision for health care must include all members of the interdisciplinary team. Nursing as a collective, representing the largest segment of the healthcare workforce, must build a structure to engage in this decision making process and hold themselves responsible to the goals of the business and consumer expectations.

A nursing shared vision also requires that nurse leaders form a new frame of reference. Nursing as a discipline facilitates successful outcomes for the business and the consumer by focusing on the point of care and leading with excellence in practice. The manager's role is to coach, mentor, and grow nurse leaders from direct care practitioners. Together they build a structure of governance to ensure that a level of professional autonomy occurs and is consistently maintained. Nurse–patient partnerships will develop and increase levels of customer satisfaction and loyalty and employee commitment (Aiken, Sochalski, & Lake, 1997).

Management must decide to resource the governance structure before any shared decision making process can occur. It is through the shared decision making process of management and staff meeting together to review strategic and quality data that leads the staff to take ownership of clinical decisions. Ownership implies a commitment to carry out the decisions at the point of care and thereby improve clinical outcomes. This is shared leadership, as illustrated in Figure 4-1.

Peer review integration is no different. Management must take an active role in facilitating the work of the staff to understand and commit to peer review. Integrating peer review into the shared governance structure should be the autonomous work of the direct care practitioners. As managers have a different organizational role, their work is to develop and integrate their own peer review process. Advanced practice nurses (APNs) and educators must do the same, as they too have unique roles.

## Valuing the Process: Resource Allocation

Budgeting for shared governance is the responsibility of management. The manager must develop the resources and create a budget that gives value to the context of the work. Protected time for the staff, separate from nonproductive time associated with the productivity measures of caring for patients, must be allocated for the staff to feel their peer review work is valued by the organization.

The structure must also align to the interdisciplinary governance structure of the organization. Organizational structures that are already in existence, such as the medical staff peer review and interdisciplinary committee structures, need defined interfaces and intersect with the nursing shared governance structure. Nursing must participate both in the discipline-specific structures and multidisciplinary structures as they exist currently and evolve over time. The nursing governance budget must be developed to include participation at all levels, and, in addition, each council must have a budget to convene work teams and implement practice change. The governance structure must have the authority to allocate these resources to accomplish their goals.

## System Change Process: Shared Leadership

Implementation and integration of peer review into existing structures is a transformative process. From the point of view of the nursing discipline, relearning must occur. The traditional peer review structure that involves the manager gathering feedback from multiple staff members to give to the reviewee is no longer applicable because the manager is not a peer of the person being reviewed. Situating peer review within the governance structure sets the stage for significant and positive change to occur as staff own the giving and receiving of peer review feedback. This implementation includes relearning of how to actualize new communication behaviors within the entire system in order for the peer review process to be successful. This will not be without organizational noise.

In a shared governance structure, authority for the decisions about all aspects of peer review design and implementation is vested organizationally in the councils. In its early phase, it is essential to develop an organizational consensus regarding the meaning of peer review, proposed implementation, and communication strategies. New behavioral expectations, supported and hardwired into human resource documents such as job descriptions and performance appraisals, are also critical. Organizations that already have a set of shared governance bylaws will need to revisit and update these documents to adopt the principles and structure of the new peer review model. Acquiring a shared meaning of peer review in an organizational context will not be easy, but it is crucial to the successful implementation of this change. Using the structure of shared governance to facilitate the authority and decisional accountability for this overall plan will lead to an employee's sense of ownership and successful adoption.

### Implementation Challenges for Managers

Suffice it to say, the process of peer review design and implementation will be seen as extremely time consuming in a nursing discipline that is already struggling to do the basic work of nursing care. Reinforcement must occur, however, through the use of legitimate power vested in the chief nursing officer (CNO) and other administrative representatives. There can be no choice about whether or not to participate in the peer review structure and process. The only individual choices are about whether to work in this new fashion. Some turnover will occur and the CNO needs to prepare the organization for this potential reality. Nursing middle managers may agree at first that this concept of peer review is good for their staff and good for the professional discipline. However, in the early phase of implementation, nurse managers may experience some unintended consequences. In the beginning, the rules about performance evaluation and peer review elements will be confusing and less than optimal outcome can occur until all the parties learn about the new rules of engagement.

Transformational leadership requires a course of action and the ability to influence others. Leaders can use the following strategies to stimulate and foster this change:

1. Understand the personal characteristics and cultural differences of each of your staff.
2. Reinforce behaviors that have made a contribution to the unit/ organization.
3. Clearly articulate nursing and organizational strategic plans and business strategies.
4. Keep communication and information flowing in all directions. Share Knowledge!
5. Make it clear that risk taking is supported.
6. Keep negative judgments to yourself.
7. Communicate role expectations and role model support for those who challenge the status quo.
8. Create a culture of safety on the unit. Facilitate staff giving and receiving feedback to and from each other.

Another source of managerial stress is related to the work of establishing a peer review process. Managers are very accustomed to receiving feedback from superiors and giving feedback to subordinates in the traditional organizational hierarchy. Giving and receiving feedback to one another across horizontal lines of communication will be stressful at first. It will be imperative that all upper level management support and engage all their managers in the process. Defining behaviors and accountabilities of management in the new model of peer review is the Nursing Management Council's work. These behaviors become the basis for management peer review.

Decision making around performance, once controlled by management, is now a highly variable multidimensional process with everyone struggling to find the external and internal locus of control. Performance evaluation is a manager's responsibility. In addition, managers own the goals development and reward and recognition processes. In peer review, the staff owns the process of defining the standards of care and holding one another accountable. The manager gets involved in the process of performance coaching only when the peer review group identifies a pattern of care deviations by the practitioner. Table 4-1 presents the new alignment of accountabilities related to peer review.

Out of this seemingly chaotic process, there will be some issues that arise where no obvious solution is apparent. These areas will create intense dialogue between management and staff. It is at this point of decision making where creativity and innovation will emerge.

**Table 4-1.   Comparison of Managerial and Peer Review Accountabilities**

| Dimensions of the Annual Performance Review | Dimensions of Peer Review |
| --- | --- |
| Goals and accomplishments | Evidence-based practice development and peer feedback |
| Attendance/staffing/workflow issues | Clinical advancement |
| Dress code | Collaborative practice agreements |
| Human resource rules/regulations | Quality, safety, and patient satisfaction outcomes |
| The Joint Commission regulatory requirements | State/professional nursing practice-related regulations and requirements |
| Behaviors related to the organization's mission, vision and values, and job performance | Behaviors related to the nursing code of ethics, the nursing model of care, and the nursing standards of care |

### Transformational Leadership

Shifting the process of decision making for peer review to the staff requires nursing administrators who are committed, resilient, flexible, visionary, and creative. Recognizing that the work of the transformational leader is in this process will be challenging, but will lead the discipline of nursing to higher levels of autonomy and accountability.

Leading in a transformational environment is often flooded with an abundance of positive energy and movement. For inspiration during these times, the leaders need only focus on the outcomes being achieved. In seeing the face of the nurse who, when dealt a difficult practice issue, is able to resolve the conflict through a peer review process; by hearing nurses proudly describing their clinical outcomes to a group of their peers; by feeling the pride of a beginning nurse moving to the next level of development through peer recognition; and by presenting the nursing annual report written by a group of nurses describing their power and influence. These outcomes are clear indicators of the recognition of the professional discipline of nursing in action and the unique role nursing plays in the quality and safety of patient care.

This next section presents shared governance structures, guiding principles, and descriptions of a council's authority and accountability for integrating various peer review processes.

## SHARED GOVERNANCE MODELS THAT INCLUDE PEER REVIEW ACCOUNTABILITY

The formal nursing peer review process needs to be aligned with the organization's nursing shared governance structure. The following guidelines provide a framework for this to occur:

- The development of a peer review plan must be identified as a strategic goal in the Nursing Strategic Plan.
- A charter for the Nursing Peer Review process and goals needs to be defined by the nursing staff for nurses at all levels of practice.
- All nursing shared governance councils must define their work and accountabilities related to peer review.
- Defining peer review practice expectations and measuring these expectations are identified as two separate and distinct processes. Each process must be located in a different shared governance council. This ensures that there is a separation of power and a check and balance system for equity.
- Peer review must be integrated at both the organization and the unit-based shared governance council structures.
- The nursing peer review structure and quality processes must align to the organization's quality initiatives.
- The nursing peer review processes must have linkage to the medical staff and other interdisciplinary structures for collaborative practice issues.
- When critical incident reviews occur, the council should have legal peer review sanction.

Each nursing organization should design its structure for best fit in its culture using the guidelines listed previously. Because each shared governance structure is unique to the organization that designed it, a variety of contemporary models are presented. Each model illustrates the point of peer review integration. The George/Haag-Heitman model integrates peer review in all aspects of the practice by locating peer review in all shared governance models. Emphasis needs to be placed on peer review activities at both the organizational and unit level.

### Unit-Based Councils

Most peer review activities are located at the point of service. The unit-based structure in Figure 4-2 is presented as a framework for the minimal unit-based structural elements needed for peer review. It is at the point, where the care is provided that most quality and safety initiatives are implemented. Achieving quality and safety outcomes for patients becomes a routine focus for peer review. Routine reviews of the population specific aggregate data is the work of the unit-based councils.

**Figure 4-2.   The minimum unit-based shared governance structure.**

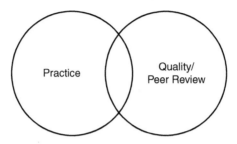

The unit-based models need linkage to the organization model for alignment and communication of point-of-care concerns. Therefore, it is imperative to design a structure utilizing the principles of peer review at the unit level that will also connect to the organizational wide councils.

The councilor model in Figure 4-3 (Porter-O'Grady, 1992) represents a conventional five council model common in the 1980s. Each council has defined authority and accountability. The peer review process is traditionally located in the Quality Council. Organizations with similar structures should examine

**Figure 4-3.   The councilor model.**

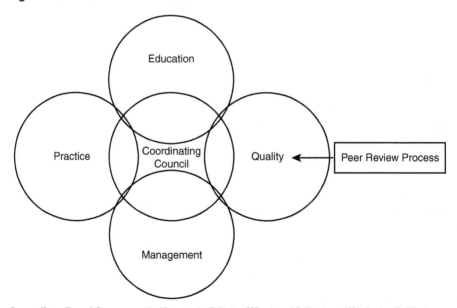

Source: From *Shared Governance for Nursing*, by T. Porter-O'Grady and S. Finnigan, 1984, Rockwell, MD: Aspen.

**Figure 4-4.   St. Luke's Medical Center model, Milwaukee, WI.**

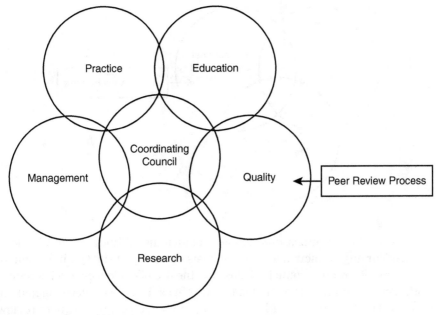

Source: Haag-Heitman, 1997

opportunities to define and locate peer review processes within the work of the other councils as well.

The model illustrated in Figure 4-4 shows the addition of the Nursing Research Council. Similar to the traditional council model, this model also locates the peer review process in the Quality Council. The contemporary model shown in Figure 4-5 integrates quality and education into a Professional Development council. As with the traditional council model, organizations should examine opportunities to define and locate peer review processes within the work of the other councils as well.

The Interdisciplinary Council structure developed by George and Haag-Heitman shown in Figure 4-6 illustrates new and innovative ways for linking and integrating interdisciplinary care. Because nursing provides care as a member of an interdisciplinary team, this structure facilitates shared decision making and communication among all the practice disciplines. Peer review is an essential component of all the discipline specific councils as each demonstrates the outcomes that contribute to the entire patient experience.

A new shared governance model that will provide for full implementation of all aspects of peer review and expands on previous models is shown in

**Figure 4-5.   The contemporary model.**

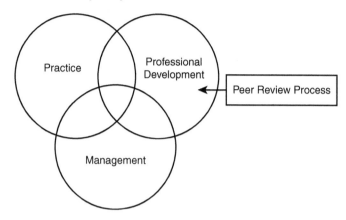

Figure 4-7. This organizational model includes the addition of an Advanced Practice Nursing council, adds an emphasis on safety in the Quality Council, and refines the practice council to illustrate the use of evidence-based practices (EBP). Peer review activities are located within each of the six decision making councils. The Nursing Executive Council (NEC) coordinates the peer review work of all the councils and aligns them to the strategic plan for nursing.

**Figure 4-6.   The interdisciplinary shared governance model.**

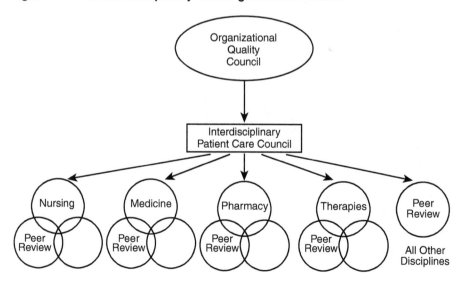

**Figure 4-7.  The fully integrated peer review model.**

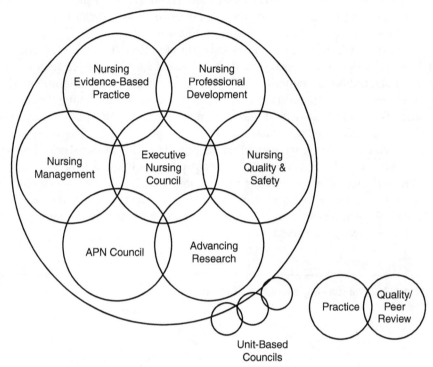

Source: © George and Haag-Heitman, 2009. Used with permission.

The peer review functions for each council are:

- Nursing Professional Development—Education and Educator Peer Review
- Nursing Quality and Safety—Clinical Care Outcomes and Staff Peer Review
- Nursing Management—Nurse Management Peer Review
- APN Council—APN Peer Review
- Nursing Evidence-Based Practice Council—Critical Incident Review
- Unit-Based Councils—Unit Peer Review

### Implementing Peer Review at the Shared Governance Councils Housewide and Unit Based

This section defines the processes for the development and implementation of shared governance structures for peer review. A redesign of current shared governance structures to reflect current practice and incorporated peer review is proposed. The accountabilities for decision making, including peer review, for each specific council is illustrated.

### Organizational Shared Governance Model

The George/Haag-Heitman governance model contains all of the essential elements to achieve nursing excellence in an organization. A description of each council's accountability and membership follows.

The use of a facilitator or outside consultant helps to expedite the process and can provide the necessary written document for the team to review. The nursing strategic plan should include the goals and identify alignment with the responsible shared governance council. The overall time frame for accomplishing the goals is identified. Each council creates a work plan to meet the goals, along with timelines associated with each process step. The appropriate nursing shared governance council chair reports on his or her work plan and progresses toward the goals at each executive council meeting.

A description of each council's accountability and membership is included. Note that there are a variety of effective shared governance models in existence. Each organization must design a model that fits with its organizational culture, resources, and goals.

---

**Figure 4-8.   The nursing executive council.**

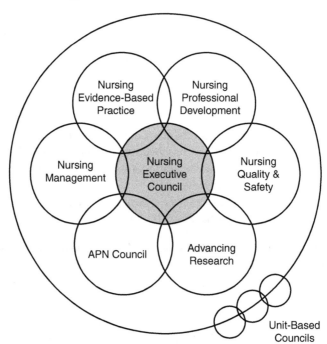

## COUNCIL DESCRIPTIONS

### The Nursing Executive Council (see Figure 4-8)

The role of the NEC is to coordinate the work of all the councils and deliver results from the strategic plan.

#### *Development of a Strategic Plan for Nursing*

As with any major change in an organizational context, one must have a plan to orchestrate the change in the most meaningful way possible. Therefore, inclusion of all levels of nursing in developing the nursing discipline strategic plan is the key to its successful implementation. This process should also include a measurement tool, timeline, and list of accountabilities assigned to each of the governance councils. The framework for content could follow the Magnet or Pathway component, especially if the plan includes a goal to accomplish getting either of those awards for the organization. In addition, the CNO should provide the organizational strategic plan to ensure alignment of the discipline plan to the organizational goals. This can also be an organizing framework especially if the organization uses a specific tool for strategic planning. The work can be accomplished in a one- to two-day retreat where all members of the nursing council and the nurses' executive team meet. There usually are other invited guests as deemed necessary for the work. For example, if there is a school of nursing aligned to the nursing discipline, then inviting the dean or faculty representative may be key to aligning the school's plan to the nursing plan. Sare and Ogilvie (2010) have written a resource specifically for strategic planning for nurses.

#### *The Nursing Executive Council Purpose*

The NEC mediates any conflict that arises between the councils. The CNO is an Executive Council member responsible for ensuring the shared governance budget is developed by requiring each council chair to submit a council budget. At the meetings, the CNO reports any system-wide issues that may impact nursing and provides updates on new goals and strategic initiatives for the organization. The Executive Council keeps appraised of regulatory changes and any new work that emerges outside the strategic plan. The councils assigns the new work to the appropriate councils for action and implementation. The NEC ensures budget allocation of resources to conduct the annual strategic planning retreat.

Membership: 7 to 15 members including the CNO, shared governance council chairs, and staff support personnel as decided by design team as stated in the bylaws.

Meeting times: Monthly for 2 hours.

Chair/chair elect: The person is elected from council membership; is responsible for setting meeting agendas; and is the contact for communication with nursing councils and other interested parties. He or she ensures Robert's Rules of Order are followed. The CNO is not necessarily the chairperson of this council.

Term: 2 years for elected members, one term reelected.

Process facilitator: He or she facilitates adherence to the agenda, acts as timekeeper, and other process issues. Often selected within group but could come from outside of the membership.

Secretary: He or she records minutes, posts agenda, facilitates communication.

Peer review: He or she is in charge of the accomplishment of the strategic planning goals and outcomes and annual reporting to the Board of Trustees.

### The Nursing Management Council (see Figure 4-9)

Purpose: To set policy and direction within the areas of management responsibility. Ensures a consistent peer review mechanism is in place for managers. Reviews management research and professional organizational literature to ensure all administrative policies, procedures, and standards of administrative

**Figure 4-9.  The nursing management council.**

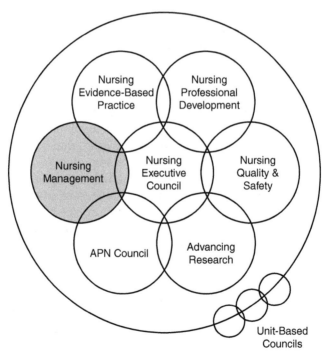

practice are evidence based. Decisions made in this group, like decisions in all shared governance councils, are final and cannot be vetoed.

Membership: 7 to 15 members. Note that when numbers of managers and directors exceeds 15 persons, then a group representing all levels of nursing leadership is elected from within the management group.

Meeting times: Monthly for 4 hours.

Chair/chair elect: Elected from council membership. Is a member of the NEC. Is responsible for setting meeting agendas and chairing meetings. Is the contact for communication with nursing councils and other interested parties. Ensures Robert's Rules of Order are followed.

Term: 2 years for elected members, one term reelected.

Process facilitator: Facilitates adherence to the agenda, acts as timekeeper and other process issues. Often selected within group but could come from outside of the membership.

Secretary: Records minutes, posts agenda, facilitates communication.

Peer review: Review allocated resources for appropriateness of use. Review of turnover and vacancy rates by unit. Review all staff satisfaction results by unit. Review all hours per patient day by unit. Review patient population specific specialty organizations standards for staffing. Review unit goal accomplishments to the strategic plan. Review distribution of all resources for reward and recognition strategies.

### Nursing Management Role Responsibilities

The manager must be able to demonstrate the skills necessary to do this work both as an elected official on the management council and in one's own role as leader. These skills include:

- Human Resource Allocation: Hiring decisions using direct care nurses in the peer interviewing process;
- Fiscal Resources: Budget planning, and dollar allocation both operating and capital;
- Material Resources: Purchasing equipment and supplies to do the work;
- System Linkages: Connecting to other departments and divisions to secure resources and flow of information, and maintaining equity within the system and discipline;
- Goal-Setting Processes: Setting performance goals to facilitate the implementation of council's decisions; and
- Reward and Recognition Strategies: The celebration of achievement.

### Important Considerations for the Essential Role of the Manager

The manager/director must be willing to share in the leadership of both the division and the unit. The manager's role is critical to staff engagement.

The manager's role should never be eliminated or consolidated because of implementation of a shared governance structure. The leader of a division or unit is more essential in the process of shared decision making as he or she becomes the coach for shared governance implementation. The role simply changes from director and controller to coach, mentor, and facilitator. The manager must support the staff in the role of decision making by coaching them in their decisional role and teaching them the processes of shared decision making. This is an important element at the unit level where 90% of all decisions take place.

**The Evidence-Based Practice Council (see Figure 4-10)**

Purpose: The EBP council defines the parameters around professional practice standards, the model of care, the behaviors of the practitioner for professional practice for advancement, the goals for consistency in clinical practice, and position descriptions of nurses and those to whom they delegate. Invested in this council are the powers necessary to make the key decisions that will impact the whole discipline of nursing as it defines clinical practice and the

---

**Figure 4-10.  The evidence-based practice council.**

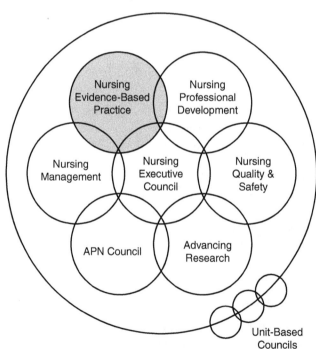

issues that affect it. Decisions made in this group, like decisions in all shared governance councils, are final and cannot be vetoed.

Membership: 7 to 15 members of nursing direct care staff selected by a nomination process or elected from the membership of the discipline organization (membership is granted to all RNs who join the organization regardless of reporting relationship to the nursing department). Consider the organization's librarian as an ad hoc member. The members will represent the discipline of nursing, not their respective areas of clinical practice.

Meeting times: Usually monthly for 4 hours.

Chair/chair elect: Elected from council membership. Is a member of the NEC. Is responsible for setting meeting agendas and chairing meetings. Is the contact for communication with nursing councils and other interested parties. Ensures Robert's Rules of Order Revised are followed.

Term: 2 years for elected members, one term reelected.

Process facilitator: Facilitates adherence to the agenda, acts as timekeeper and other process issues. Often selected within the group but could come from outside the membership.

Secretary: Records minutes, posts agenda, facilitates communication.

Peer Review: Ensures the use of peer reviewed journals for EBP application. Reviews all clinical policies and procedures for EBP foundation. Ensures all unit councils are applying the principles of the model of care. Reviews all critical incidents for action.

### Nursing Quality and Safety Council (see Figure 4-11)

Purpose: Develops the nursing quality and safety plan and sets the annual goals for nursing discipline quality outcomes. Monitors the quality dashboard and governs the unit-based council activity in achieving outcomes and benchmarks for the quality goals. Defines peer review processes and measurement for quality and safety at the housewide, unit, and individual levels. Receives recommendations from EBP council on practice changes from critical incident reviews that must be measured and evaluated for outcomes.

Membership: 7 to 15 members of nursing direct care staff selected by a nomination process or elected from the membership of the discipline organization (membership is granted to all RNs who join the organization regardless of reporting relationship to nursing department). The members will represent the discipline of nursing, not their respective areas of clinical practice. Ad hoc members: Nursing and hospital quality representatives, risk managers, and safety officer.

Meeting times: Monthly for 4 hours.

Chair/chair elect: Elected from council membership. Is a member of the NEC. Is responsible for setting meeting agendas and chairing meetings. Is the

**Figure 4-11. The nursing quality and safety council.**

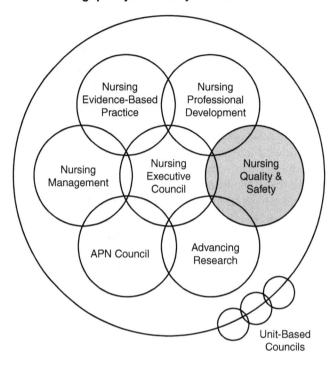

contact for communication with nursing councils and other interested parties. Ensures Robert's Rules of Order are followed.

Term: 2 years for elected members, one term reelected.

Process facilitator: Facilitates adherence to the agenda, acts as timekeeper, and other process issues. Often selected within group but could come from outside of the membership.

Secretary: Records minutes, posts agenda, facilitates communication.

Peer review: Holds each unit accountable to the quality dashboard outcomes. Evaluates the peer review process at the organization and unit level.

### Nursing Professional Development Council (see Figure 4-12)

Purpose: To develop education programs and educational needs assessment. Reviews research and evidence-based educational models to ensure flexibility for individual learning styles. Reviews and approves the nursing professional education and travel budget. Plans annual nursing day celebration in collaboration with Nursing Management Council. Oversees and governs all orientation and residency programs for clinical staff including preceptor training and

**Figure 4-12.   The nursing professional development council.**

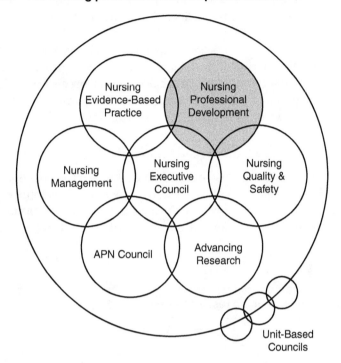

evaluation. Develops evaluation and review processes for education programming. Coordinates with schools of nursing for clinical placement. Governs
the unit-based approach to all of the above responsibilities. Establishes the
process for evaluation of all peer review of clinical development advancement
programs.

Membership: 7 to 15 members of nursing direct care staff selected by a
nomination process or elected from the membership of the discipline organization (membership is granted to all RNs who join the organization regardless
of reporting relationship to nursing department). The members will represent
the discipline of nursing, not their respective areas of clinical practice. Ad hoc
membership: Nursing education director/manager, school of nursing representatives, and HR or other organizational development representatives.

Meeting times: Monthly for 4 hours.

Chair/chair elect: Elected from council membership. Is a member of the
NEC. Is responsible for setting meeting agendas and chairing meetings. Is the
contact for communication with nursing councils and other interested parties.
Ensures Robert's Rules of Order are followed.

Term: 2 years for elected members, one term reelected.

Process facilitator: Facilitates adherence to the agenda, acts as timekeeper, and other process issues. Often selected within group but could come from outside of the membership.

Secretary: Records minutes, posts agenda, facilitates communication.

Peer review: Evaluation of the educational programs provided at the organization and unit level. Evaluation of the orientation, preceptor, and residency programs. Evaluation of school of nursing clinical experiences. Evaluation of the professional development advancement program.

### Advancing Research Council (see Figure 4-13)

Purpose: Sets the nursing research agenda. Chooses the conceptual framework model for research. Validates new knowledge development. Tracks and trends all nursing research performed in the organization. Maintains a relationship with Institutional Review Board (IRB). Develops, a nursing

**Figure 4-13.  The advancing research council.**

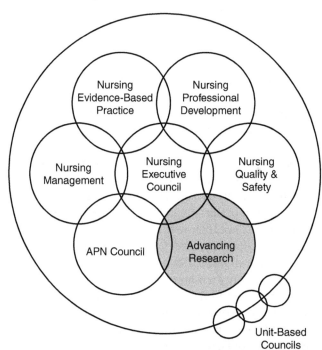

scholars' program to foster direct care nurse involvement in research where appropriate.

Membership: 7 to 15 members of direct care nurses and APNs staff and the Director of Research and EBP. Selected by a nomination process or elected from the membership of the discipline organization (membership is granted to all RNs who join the organization regardless of reporting relationship to nursing department). The members will represent the discipline of nursing, not their respective areas of clinical practice. Ad hoc membership: Nursing education director/manager, school of nursing representatives, PhD in nursing research (if consultant), and librarian.

Meeting times: Monthly for 2 hours.

Chair/chair elect: Elected from council membership. Is a member of the NEC. Is responsible for setting meeting agendas and chairing meetings. Is the contact for communication with nursing councils and other interested parties. Ensures Robert's Rules of Order are followed.

Term: 2 years for elected members, one term reelected.

Process facilitator: Facilitates adherence to the agenda, acts as timekeeper, and other process issues. Often selected within group but could come from outside of the membership.

Secretary: Records minutes, posts agenda, facilitates communication.

Peer review: Annual measurement of nursing research agenda. Ensures unit level adoption of the model for research. Reviews all internal and external nursing research projects.

## Advanced Practice Council (see Figure 4-14)

Purpose: Defines the accountabilities for all APNs in the organization as it relates to the discipline of nursing. Requires ongoing review of APN practice standards, policies, and processes of national and state credentialing and licensing programs. Provides consultation regarding APN practice-related issues within the organization. Advances APN practice.

Membership: 7 to 15 APNs; selected by a nomination process or elected from the membership of the discipline organization (membership is granted to all APNs who join the organization regardless of reporting relationship to the nursing department). The members will represent the discipline of nursing, not their respective areas of clinical practice.

Meeting times: Monthly for 2 hours.

Chair/chair elect: Elected from council membership. Is a member of the NEC. Is responsible for setting meeting agendas and for chairing meetings. Is the contact for communication with nursing councils and other interested parties. Ensures Robert's Rules of Order are followed.

Term: 2 years for elected members, one term reelected.

**Figure 4-14.  The APN council.**

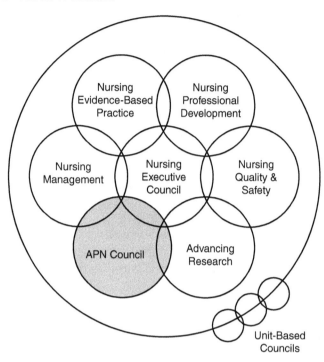

Process facilitator: Facilitates adherence to the agenda, acts as timekeeper and other process issues. Often selected within group but could come from outside of the membership.

Secretary: Records minutes, posts agenda, facilitates communication.

Peer review: Establishes a formal peer review process for the APN roles. Reviews case studies for quality outcomes. Reviews all APN credentials and reviews all new APN privilege requests.

### Accomplishing Nursing Council Work Through the Use of Commissioned Work Groups

Each council has the authority to delegate special projects and areas of concern to time-limited work groups. Work groups perform specific tasks and scopes of work that are delegated by a council, and are recommending bodies, not decisional groups. They receive their purpose, membership (use of experts for content recommendations), timeline for the work, and the scope of the deliverables required from the delegating nursing council. Each council should budget for work groups based on next year's assignments from the strategic plan.

### Standing Committees

Committees are designed and developed by the council they report to, are nondecisional, and have regular members and meet on a consistent basis. The chair is usually a member of the respective council that has chartered the work. The committee membership's time must be budgeted by the nursing council to whom they report and from whom they take their assignment. Examples might include Policy and Procedure Committee, Clinical Advancement Review Committee, and Clinical/IT Documentation Committee.

### Unit-Based Shared Governance

Unit-based shared governance councils are important components of the entire shared governance process. It is at the unit base or point of service that 90% of all practice decisions are implemented.

### Structure

The structure needs to respond to the service demand and work culture of the unit. It is essential that every work unit applies the prevailing principles of shared governance and that there is a clear communication path for nursing issues from unit to unit and unit to the organizational councils. Each unit-based council must align to the organizational goals as illustrated in Figure 4-15.

### Unit-Based Models

Membership: A majority of direct care RNs, along with a manager, APN, educator, and other roles as applicable. In some cases unit membership is limited by the number of RNs in each unit. The concept of clustering representatives from similar units is used. It is essential to identify the representative from clustered units to the housewide governance councils. Clustering unit members assume authority for ensuring each unit complies with expectations and obligations.

Meeting times: Monthly for 4 hours.

Chair/chair elect: Direct care RNs chair all councils at the unit level. Elected from council membership. Is responsible for setting meeting agendas

---

**Figure 4-15. The unit-based councils.**

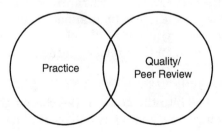

and chairing meetings. Is the contact for communication with nursing councils and other interested parties. Ensures Robert's Rules of Order are followed.

Term: 2 years for elected members, one term reelected.

Process Facilitator: Facilitates adherence to the agenda, acts as time keeper, and other process issues. Often selected within group but could come from outside of the membership.

Secretary: Records minutes, posts agenda, facilitates communication.

### Practice Council Peer Review Accountabilities

- Standards development/evidence-based practice
- Job descriptions
- Clinical advancement programs
- Research
- Unit education plan
- Individual education plan
- Patient-based education plan
- Unit orientation plan
- New technology or practice education
- Education for practice deficiency

### Quality Council Peer Review Accountabilities

- Interdisciplinary concerns
- Quality and safety initiatives
- Peer review credentialing and privileging
- Corrective measures and actions
- Attendance at professional staff meetings

## Measuring Successful Outcomes

### Peer Review Evaluation

Evaluation of each element of the peer review process is necessary following the initial implementation process. The shared governance councils are responsible for this evaluation, assuring input from all stakeholder groups to assure the goals of the peer review process are met. An example of an evaluation is provided below for the role actualization aspect of peer review. In this example, the nurse receiving the review completes the feedback form and submits to the Quality Council for their review and action.

### Enhancing Quality and Safety Outcomes

Integrating peer review into the goals of the shared governance councils drives improvement in quality and safety outcomes. These improvements will be apparent in the individual-, unit-, and organization-wide performance metrics. Upon meeting both organizational and unit benchmarks, the organization- and unit-based practice councils can identify additional targets to advance the practice using new and emerging evidence-based practice knowledge and research.

### Shared Leadership Outcomes

Shared leadership of an empowered workforce, facilitated through the shared governance structure and processes, are reflected in the enhanced staff engagement and ownership of role accountabilities. From participation in the shared governance structure and the shared decision-making process, each participant experiences shared leadership. The shared balance of power between managers and staff can result in the following outcomes.

Each participant learns to:

- Trust in the team and integrity of the organizational and professional commitment to its mission, vision, and values.
- Invest in the continued development of the point-of-service workforce, recognizing that he or she is the organization's most valuable resource. A positive business outcome is realized as a result of this investment.
- Value and reward the contributions of both individuals and team achievements as defined by the outcomes of established quality and safety goals and targets.
- Understand the importance of team learning and the value of collaborative efforts. As the parts of the system come together as a whole, silos are broken, encouraging risk taking, addressing sacred cows that impede practice, and setting up the conditions for creativity and innovation.
- Partner with all members of the healthcare team and value the shared governance principles of partnership, equity, ownership, and accountability. This partnership extends to each customer, patient, and family and is displayed in patient satisfaction and loyalty scores.
- Effectively participate in the shared decision-making process and to develop a deep appreciation for skilled leadership behaviors for all organizational roles.
- Successfully use the peer review to improve patient safety, the quality of care, and the care provider in a just culture.

As the culture shifts with new models of shared decision making in nursing and point of service, employees are recognized in new ways for their contributions to patient and organizational outcomes, members of the interdisciplinary professional team will take note. Organizations can anticipate that when nursing empowerment becomes visible to other disciplines in the organization, inquiry about an interdisciplinary shared governance structure may emerge, as illustrated in Figure 4-6. This milestone is indicative of a cultural transformation to an empowered workplace.

A comparison of leadership behaviors found in the literature (Manning & Curtis, 2003; Rosen & Brown, 1996; Vogt & Murrell, 1990) and practice according to the level of organizational empowerment is illustrated in Table 4-2.

**Table 4-2.  Comparison of Leadership Behaviors According to the Level of Organizational Empowerment**

| Leadership Behaviors | Hierarchic Management (Not empowered) | Unbalanced and Disorganized Environment | Empowered, Professional Environment |
|---|---|---|---|
| **Decision Making** | Leader makes all decisions. | No one is clear on decisions. | Staff own staff decisions regarding their roles and responsibilities and partners with management in shared responsibilities. |
| **Performance Evaluation** | Leader decides the plan and reviews with subordinate. | There is no performance plan. | Staff engage in self-assessment and identify their goals prior to review with manager. |
| **Policy Making** | Leader decides all policy and authorizes all changes. | Staff and managers often act confused about or do not consistently follow policies. | Staff decide practice policy. Management decides administrative policy. |
| **Problem Solving** | Wait and see behavior by workers; expectation for management to fix all problems. | Lack of problem-solving framework and identification of authority and locus of control, leading to decisions being made in more than one place. | Staff and management partner to resolve problems and seek alternative solutions. |
| **Taking Initiative** | Employees wait to be assigned work and do not volunteer. | Lack of communication about initiatives and no consistent process for communication. | Recognition of solutions and action taking to resolve. Employees see it and own it. |

| | | | |
|---|---|---|---|
| **Defining Roles** | Roles and responsibilities are defined by leader. | Confusion regarding roles and authority for decision making. | All roles are clearly defined along with accountabilities. |
| **Setting Standards** | The leader defines and sets all standards. | Lack of consistent application of practice standards. | Professionals define and implement their unique clinical standards and partner with management to define organizational behavioral standards. |
| **Peer Review Process** | The leader decides and implements the framework for peer review process. | Leader collects peer feedback for each employee and anonymously delivers this feedback to employees. | Clinical staff define their peer review framework and implement it for all clinical roles. Management defines and implements their role-specific peer review process. |

## LEADING INTO THE FUTURE

The business success of the future of health care rests with the understanding of the executive leadership that all employees, especially those at the point of service, possess important personal and professional knowledge about the impact of their role on the outcomes of patients. Leveraging this wisdom is one essential strategy for organizational success. Creating mechanisms to continually access this knowledge and use it to advance the work of the organization requires new partnerships and abandoning the hierarchic top-down approach that is entrenched in many healthcare organizations. Frequent two way, face-to-face communication sessions with all employees enhances employee engagement and provides important insights about the impact of business decisions. While this may go without saying, but in many organizations, e-mails, bulletin boards, and messages placed on the back of the bathroom door, frequently replace human interactions.

Assuring that managers are routinely present at unit-based council meetings is one strategy to enhance communication, organizational alignment, and shared leadership. The consistent attendance of elected managerial representatives on organization-wide councils is also important. The manager's role at the council meetings is not to direct and control, but rather to hear the discussions and understand the meaning of issues from staff perspectives. The manager facilitates decision making through the sharing of knowledge of additional resources and perspectives, and by helping to make system linkages into the decision-making process.

The empowered workplace is further facilitated by building clear role definitions and accountabilities throughout the organization, and by building a whole system structure for all employees to participate. Engaging all employees to achieve the strategic initiatives of the organization is enhanced by translating organization goals into individual and unit-level goals. Resourcing the means to achieve these initiatives is an important role of management. Creating the conditions for an empowered workplace advances employee engagement and their freedom to act and assist the organization in achieving its long-term mission. Employee-driven problem solving is a powerful alternative to expectations of management to fixes to problems. Recognizing and rewarding new and preferred behaviors is essential to maintain this cultural change.

Achieving quality and safety outcomes across disciplines follows that same path as nursing. Regardless of discipline, all professional staff own all aspects of the self-regulation process, including their discipline-specific peer review, and, as professionals, have the same authority to govern over those decisions as necessary. The interdisciplinary shard governance structure illustrated in Figure 4-6 is the structure to integrate peer review for all disciplines based on the standards of care  and  the evidence-based practices of the discipline. With implementation of peer review and shared governane, the work of restructring the health care environment around the principles of partnership, equity ownership, and accountability is complete.

## REFERENCES

Aiken, L. H., Sochalski, J., & Lake, E. T. (1997). Studying outcomes of organizational change in health services. *Medical Care, 35*, NS6–N18.

American Nurses Association. (1988). *Peer review in nursing practice*. Kansas City, MO: Author.

Boyett, J. H., & Conn, H. D. (1991). *Workplace 2000: The revolution reshaping American business*. New York, NY: Plume.

Donabedian, A. (1988). The quality of care how it can be assessed? *Journal of the American Medical Association, 260*(12), 1743–1748

Kanter, R. M. (1979). *Men and women of the corporation*. New York, NY: Basic Books.

Manning, G. & Curtis, K. (2003). *The art of leadership*. Boston: McGraw-Hill Irwin.

Porter-O'Grady, T. (1992). Implementing shared governance: creating a professional organization. Baltimore, MD: Mosby.

Rosen, R, & Brown, P. (1996). *Leading people: Transforming business from inside out*. New York: Viking.

Sare, M. V., & Ogilvie, L. (2010). *Strategic planning for nurses: Change management for health care*. Sudbury, MA: Jones and Bartlett.

Vogt, J., & Murrell, K. (1990). *Empowerment in organizations*. San Diego: University Associates.

# CHAPTER 5

# Guiding Principles, Practices, and Organizational Alignment

*Without change there is no innovation, creativity, or incentive for*
*improvement. Those who initiate change will have a better opportunity to*
*manage the change that is inevitable.*

— WILLIAM POLLARD

An assortment of shared governance structures and council descriptions are provided in Chapter 4. More detail on the integration of peer review activities into the shared governance structure is provided here, along with contemporary peer review principles for application in all peer review procedures. The American Nurses' Association (ANA) Peer Review Guidelines (1988) outlined important principles and tenets making peer review essential for the advancement of the profession of nursing. The following excerpts from the 1988 publication provide the groundwork of contemporary peer review principles and practices:

Nurses who carry the authority and responsibility for implementing the peer review program provide a unique and vital service on behalf of patients, families, the community, their nursing colleagues, and the institution, agency, or other setting in which they work. In serving all these constituencies, they serve the profession as a whole.

Peer reviewers are nurse colleagues with clinical competence similar to that of the nurse seeking peer review. Nurse reviewers need, or must strive to develop, the judicial temperament—the capacity and the willingness to make critical decisions on the basis of evidence. A constructive approach is important in rendering judgments. Feedback to the nurse under review is most effective when both verbal and written communication are combined. This collegial process can be carried on with security in the knowledge that quantity of care, however extensive, and cost of care, however contained, lose meaning unless the quality of that care is professionally affirmed.

The steps in the process of peer review are the same for all nurses and all settings. The key difference lies in identifying the purpose, the peer group, and the appropriate professionally defined standards upon which to base the review. The peer review program must provide for confidentiality with regard to patient care records and must honor the rights of the nurses being reviewed, the reviewers, the clients, the nurse administrators, and other professionals who share responsibility for patient care.

Individuals, institutions, and the nursing profession all derive benefits from an effective peer review program. With respect to the individual, participation in the peer review process stimulates professional growth. Clinical knowledge and skills are updated. Within the institution, effective peer review points towards changes in educational and administrative patterns needed to ensure quality, and it reveals opportunities for research pertinent to the enhancement of practice. As to the professional as a whole, improved quality of care by individuals and agencies, accompanied by self-regulation of nursing practice, can only serve to strengthen nursing. (ANA, 1988, pp. 4–14)

## CONTEMPORARY PEER REVIEW PRINCIPLES

The application of peer review principles creates a different context for operating and functioning in the organization and will alter the relational milieu. Management requests around peer input at the time of the annual performance review will no longer be the hub of peer review activities. A new focus on the need for horizontal relationships and peer partnerships to attain quality and safety outcomes along the continuum of care will emerge. Sustained achievement of the desired outcomes begins with a new meaning of peer review and a principled approach. These set of principles exemplify peer review rather than simply defining it. As with other emerging healthcare structures and models, and the move into a new age of understanding and application, the ability to discern is better than the ability to define (Porter-O'Grady, 2009). The following six principles are presented to guide thinking about the foundations for action and serve as a template for measuring the consistency between actions and beliefs:

1. A peer is someone of the same rank.
2. Peer review is practice focused.
3. Feedback is timely, routine, and a continuous expectation.
4. Peer review fosters a continuous learning culture of patient safety and best practice.
5. Feedback is not anonymous.
6. Feedback incorporates the developmental stage of the nurse.

As illustrated in Table 5-1, these six principles stem from and are grounded in the 1988 ANA guidelines. The impact of these peer review principles can be dramatic in changing the professional practice environment. Each has its unique characteristics and features.

### Principle #1: A peer is someone of the same rank.

Much of the distrust and misunderstanding that nurses have about peer review comes no doubt from the misguided notion that peer review is a managerial process. For most organizations, the only formal process to capture peer feedback is related

**Table 5-1.  Evolution of Contemporary Peer Review with 1988 ANA Guidelines**

| Six Contemporary Peer Review Principles | 1988 ANA Guidelines |
| --- | --- |
| 1. A peer is someone of the same rank. | Peer review implies that the nursing care delivered by a group of nurses or an individual nurse is evaluated by individuals of the same rank or standing according to established standards of practice. |
| | Peer reviewers are nurse colleagues with clinical competence similar to that of the nurse seeking peer review. |
| | The steps in the process of peer review are the same for all nurses and all settings. |
| | The key difference lies in identifying the purpose, the peer group, and the appropriate professionally defined standards upon which to base the review. |
| 2. Peer review is practice focused. | Standards of nursing practice provide a means for measuring the quality of nursing care a client receives. |
| | Peer review in nursing is the process by which practicing registered nurses systematically access, monitor, and make judgments about the quality of nursing care provided by peers as measured against professional standards of practice. |
| | Peer review activities are focused on the practice decisions of professional nurses to determine the appropriateness and timeliness of those decisions. |
| 3. Feedback is timely, routine, and a continuous expectation. | In every healthcare facility in which nurses practice and for each nurse in individual practice, provision for peer review should be an ongoing process. |
| | An organized program makes peer review timely and objective. |
| 4. Peer review fosters a continuous learning culture of patient safety and best practice. | The goals of every agency providing nursing care should include peer review as one means of maintaining standards of nursing practice and upgrading nursing care. |
| | With respect to the individual, participation in the peer review process stimulates professional growth. Clinical knowledge and skills are updated. |

*(continues)*

**Table 5-1.    Evolution of Contemporary Peer Review with 1988 ANA Guidelines**
**(Continued)**

| Six Contemporary Peer Review Principles | 1988 ANA Guidelines |
|---|---|
| | The purposes of peer review are to determine the strengths and weaknesses of nursing care, taking into consideration local and institutional resources and constraints; to provide evidence for use as the basis of recommendations for new or altered policies and procedures to improve nursing care; and to identify those areas where practice patterns indicate more knowledge is needed. |
| | Nurse reviewers need, or must strive to develop, the judicial temperament, the capacity and the willingness, to make critical decisions on the basis of evidence. |
| 5. Feedback is not anonymous. | Feedback to the nurse under review is most effective when both verbal and written communication are combined. |
| 6. Feedback incorporates the developmental stage of the nurse. | Individuals, institutions, and the nursing profession all derive benefits from an effective peer review program. With respect to the individual, participation in the peer review process stimulates professional growth. Clinical knowledge and skills are updated. |

to the performance evaluation procedure. This misconception stems from the managerial practice of obtaining peer input for the annual performance review and then summarizing and presenting this feedback to the reviewee, usually without identifying the sources of the peer input. Eliminating this obstacle to progress will require that all nurses recognize the inadequacy of this practice in achieving quality outcomes and realign with their peer group for authentic peer review.

Establishing clear boundaries and definitions about the peer groups is essential in creating effective peer review processes. It is important to note that managers are not peers with direct care nurses even though they have practiced as direct care nurses. Appropriate peer groups include:

- Direct care nurse to direct care nurse
- Advanced practice nurse (APN) to APN
- Educator to educator
- Manager to manager
- Director to director
- Chief nursing officer (CNO) to CNO

As a result of this reality, peer review practices for the CNO need to be forged.

**Principle #2: Peer review is practice focused.**

The evidence-based, safety- and quality-driven culture of health care today has created the need for all roles to ensure their functionality, cost-effectiveness, and service orientation. "The demand for outcomes (value) ultimately focuses on the performance of those upon whom outcomes depend" (Porter-O'Grady, 2009, p. 21). A new focus on the contribution that each role has on the achievement of professional and organization outcomes is needed. The healthcare environment has been laden with an upsurge of regulatory quality and safety standards. Nursing has also experienced an expansion in the role-based standards for nurses across all practice roles and specialties. Peer review provides the mechanism to ensure that these new standards are addressed and new roles are achieving their intended outcomes. Effective peer review incorporates nationally recognized, evidence-based practice, and quality and safety standards with an emphasis on the outcomes of these practices.

**Principle #3: Feedback is timely, routine, and a continuous expectation.**

Nursing is practiced within a complex social system that defines the rules, norms, values, and role expectations within the culture. An open exchange of information and feedback is essential for this social system to survive and thrive. Feedback from external sources, such as regulatory bodies, causes internal reactions in the healthcare environment. Traditionally, reaction to the external feedback has been done by management, often resulting in practice mandates being handed down to the point-of-service providers in a hierarchic fashion. Experience has demonstrated the ineffectiveness of this top-down approach and the need for shared decision making using the shared governance structure. Feedback also occurs as an internal process resulting from actions within the social system itself. Patient satisfaction and employee engagement are both examples of internal feedback mechanisms.

Whether internal or external, the value of feedback is in its potential to create disequilibrium and set up the conditions for new learning. Achieving continuous quality improvements demands that organizations create cultures that support dynamic open-system feedback at all levels of the organization, starting at the point of service. Therefore, peer feedback needs to be timely, continuous, and a routine expectation. Moving from a traditional static process to continuous and "just-in-time" expectations creates feedback that is fast, fluid, flexible, and responsive to the desired outcomes.

Nurses at East Jefferson General Hospital in Metairie, Louisiana, discovered the value of just-in-time feedback in achieving outcomes that their other focused efforts could not. They reported,

> In striving to improve the accuracy of the patient discharge home medication list, our team implemented many strategies, including quality management nurse audits,

feedback from supervisors, numerous "hot tips" and adjustments to the computer-ized system. All of our efforts were met with little success until we incorporated practice-focused, just-in-time, meaningful feedback from one staff nurse to another. (Courtesy of East Jefferson General Hospital. Metairie, LA. All rights reserved.)

A full description of their quality approach to improve the accuracy of the medication reconciliation process can be found in Appendix B.

### Principle #4: Peer review fosters a continuous learning culture of patient safety and best practice.

Effective peer review must be conducted in the framework of a learning organi-zation and just culture. A focused systems approach using double loop learning is needed to completely identify system issues that hamper quality and safety initiatives. Traditionally, errors in nursing have often been dealt with in unsys-tematic, punitive, and ineffective means, with little knowledge of the factors influencing error generation (Anderson & Webster, 2001). By blaming or focus-ing on the individual, contributing factors will not be uncovered, and a sense of blame and shame is created. A collective understanding of these contributing factors is important in creating a just culture and moving away from person-centered blame that views unsafe acts as arising from carelessness, neglect, forgetfulness, inattention, and poor motivation. Peer review can provide the means for an effective systems-centered approach to error reduction, as real-ized by other high-risk industries such as aviation, and nuclear power.

A continuous learning culture shifts the focus from individual learning to organizational learning and helps foster a common commitment to achieve and sustain desired outcomes. In addition to the detection and correction of errors, a continuous learning culture using double loop learning also questions the assumptions and norms about practice and helps modify these norms, including policies and procedures. Modifications in practice helps advance the practice and calls for new learning as well as unlearning of ineffective or unsafe processes.

Lifelong learning is not a new concept for nursing professionals. Our founder, Florence Nightingale, identified the essential role that lifelong learn-ing plays in practice development over a century ago.

> For us who Nurse, our Nursing is a thing, which, unless in it we are making *progress* every year, every month, every week – take my word for it we are going *back*. The more experience we gain, the more progress we can make. The prog-ress you make in your year's training with us is as nothing to what you must make every year *after* your year's training is over. A woman who thinks in herself: "Now I am a 'full' Nurse, a 'skilled' Nurse – I have learnt all that there is to be learnt"; take my word for it she does not know *what a Nurse is,* and she never will know: she is *gone* back already. (Dossey, Selanders, Beck, & Attewell, 2005, p. 31)

**Principle #5: Feedback is not anonymous.**

Anonymity is not compatible with a continuous learning culture for quality and safety. Effective team learning emerges from both dialogue and skillful discussion. Dialogue is the sustained collective inquiry into everyday, often taken for granted, experiences. Using skillful discussion, teams can see how components of the situation fit together and develop a deeper understanding of the forces at play among them (Senge, Kleiner, Roberts, Ross, & Smith, 1994). This system approach is important to understanding barriers to the achievement of quality and safety outcomes.

Many nurses feel that anonymous feedback is the only real way to obtain honest feedback, although this notion lacks empirical support. There is no evidence that anonymous feedback has ever facilitated positive professional performance or positively impacted patient care. Many nurses equate feedback with potential conflict and feel ill equipped to deliver skilled communication, preferring to give anonymous feedback when required. The notion that conflict is destructive to organizational life and interferes with workplace stability and harmony comes from the traditional management literature from the 1940s era. During this time, managers were taught to control the expression of anger at all costs (Valentine, 1995). The idea that conflict could serve positive functions by encouraging creativity did not emerge until the 1960s and 1970s (Valentine, 1995). Despite this radial shift in the way conflict was viewed, the negative connotation about conflict remains a substantial barrier to effective engagement in person-to-person feedback today.

A nurse's duty to use respectful communication with an open exchange of views to preserve practice integrity and safety is called for in the Code of Ethics for Nurses (ANA, 2001). Therefore, the use of anonymous feedback violates the Code of Ethics for Nurses and other professional standards. Along this same line, the American Association of Critical-Care Nurses (AACN) identified that deficient interpersonal skills can create a culture of silence that can harm or even kill patients. The AACN recognizes that "a culture of safety and excellence requires that individual nurses and healthcare organizations make it a priority to develop among professionals communication skills–including written, spoken and non-verbal–that are on a par with expert clinical skills" (AACN, 2005, p. 17). All participants must be able to engage in dialogue and freely ask questions and clarify information and perceptions.

**Principle #6: Feedback incorporates the developmental stage of the nurse.**

Peer feedback needs to be appropriate for identified expectations about the each nurse's expected level of problem-solving ability for clinical decision making. Decades of research informs us that developmentally, nurse's clinical judgment and decision making, caring, and collaboration practices vary along a novice-to-expert continuum (Benner, 1984; Haag-Heitman, 1999). For example, it is unfair to expect novice nurses to be able to recognize subtle, early warning signs of decline, as they reason things through analytically and must learn how to recognize a situation in which only a particular aspect of theoretical knowledge applies (Tanner, 2006). Recognizing subtle changes and initiating interventions to ward off complications takes years of experience.

Integrating peer feedback with the characteristics of practice related to the developmental stage of nurses along the novice-to-expert framework will both facilitate professional growth and inform the profession about strategies that foster development of nurses beyond the beginner level. The need to understand strategies to foster professional development is summarized: "the benefits of expert nursing practice are far-reaching, yet we know little how to promote it and what conditions foster its development" (Williams, 1996, p. iv). There is a general lack of formalized systematic approaches to foster nursing practice-based skill development and continuous learning beyond the initial orientation stages and beginner stages, despite the potential for superior outcomes associated with expert nursing performance (Almada, Carafoli, Flattery, French, & McNamara, 2004; Santucci, 2004). This widespread void of practice development programs for experienced practicing nurses is harmful to the profession, and ultimately to patient and family outcomes, and their absence underscores the notion that a graduate of an accredited school is a finished product and the fallacy that "a nurse is a nurse is a nurse" (Barnum, 1996, p. viii). Peer review has the potential to significantly help fill this gap.

## AREAS OF PEER REVIEW

In the Code of Ethics for Nurses (2001), the ANA recognized that effective peer review is indispensable to hold nursing practice to the highest standards of care and practice. Peer review helps address the boundaries of duty and loyalty for all nurses, including "the responsibility to preserve integrity and safety, to maintain competence, and to continue personal and professional growth" (ANA, 2001, p. 18). These concepts, combined with the ANA (1988) Peer Review Guidelines, focus on maintaining standards of nursing practice and upgrading nursing care in three contemporary focus areas for peer review. The three areas are: (1) quality and safety, (2) role actualization, and (3) practice advancement. Each area of contemporary peer review has an organizational, unit, and individual focus. Figure 5-1 illustrates the areas of focus for peer review.

The 1988 peer review guidelines makes recommendations on both peer review structures and procedures, including the establishment of a separate peer review committee. The evolution of professional practice environments

**Figure 5-1.    Contemporary focus on peer review.**

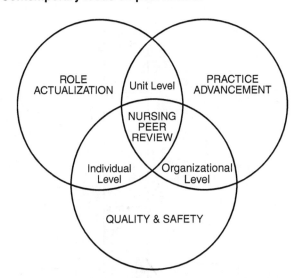

over the past several decades now more appropriately aligns peer review activities within an organization's shared governance structure, the foundational principles of which are presented in Chapter 4. A separate peer review committee is not recommended as it would violate the authority of the shared governance councils and is too limiting for all the areas needed for nursing peer review. The principles used for the peer review processes are the same for nurses in all settings with the key differences being the peer group and the appropriate professionally defined standards used. Alignment of peer review is done according to the specific focus area of peer review and the roles and accountabilities of the shared governance councils as illustrated in Figure 5-2.

## PEER REVIEW FOCUS ON QUALITY AND SAFETY

### Structure and Alignment

The Nursing Quality and Safety Council and the Nursing Management Council (NMC) have primary responsibility for setting the goals related to quality and safety for direct care nurses and management. Peer review functions of the NMC are presented later in this chapter. Substantial involvement of the Nursing Quality and Safety Council in peer review is warranted as it is responsible for evaluating and measuring the quality of nursing care and the quality of the nursing care provider. The quality movement in the United States has significantly increased the number of quality and safety initiatives across all practice

**Figure 5-2.    The organizational alignment for nursing peer review.**

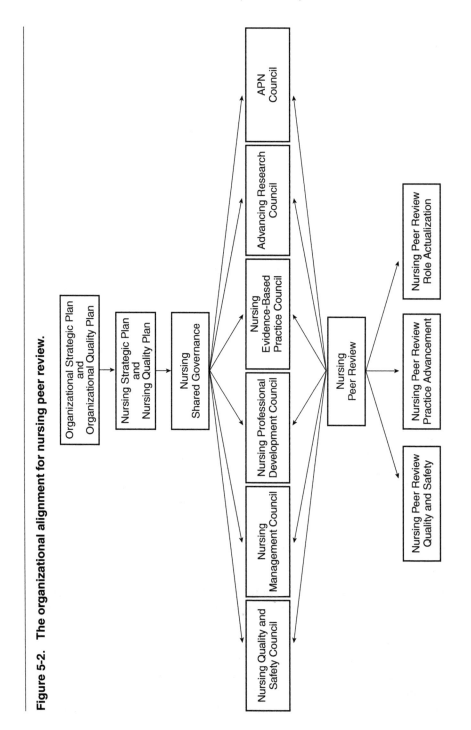

settings along with a heightened demand for obtaining results. The Nursing Quality and Safety Council's strategic initiatives form the context for nursing peer review for the organization, patient care units, and the individual nurse. These initiatives (or goals) must closely align with the hospital's Quality Council strategic objectives. Each quality goal and strategy must be clearly defined and measure the discipline specific aspects needed to achieve the goal. The unit-based shared governance councils engage in peer review by applying the organization's goals and quality measures to their unique patient populations. Progression toward goals achievement as defined by the Nursing Strategic Plan is monitored by the Nursing Executive Council.

Recognizing that quality initiatives must be driven from the point of service, the Hospital Quality Department staff provides support to the Nursing Quality and Safety Council through the development of a nursing quality scorecard or dashboard. Both organizational and unit specific quality scores for national benchmarks, such as the National Database on Nursing Quality Indicators (NDNQI), The Joint Commission (TJC), patient satisfaction data and employee satisfaction, should be included in the scorecard for comparison purposes. These scorecards and dashboards highlight specific areas that need peer review involvement to achieve identified benchmarks. The value of nursing's work is measured by the outcomes achieved and are critical to the discipline's future as the outcome data becomes the input for reports to the Boards of Trustees, regulatory groups, and to demonstrate nursing excellence for Magnet and other quality designations. Peer review substantially contributes to the achievement of nursing's strategic goals for quality and safety at the organization-, unit-, and patient-specific levels as illustrated in the following practice examples.

### The Nursing Strategic Plan Defines Quality Goals

The nursing strategic plan defines and aligns the nursing goals with the organization's goals to help ensure organizational success, resources allocation, and patient outcomes. Integrating quality activities into existing processes rather than redesigning processes greatly reduces the learning and implementation time for outcomes to be achieved (Harrington, 2009) and is consistent with the principles of shared governance. An example of a nursing strategic plan from Poudre Valley Medical Center, a Magnet hospital, with focused quality or clinical performance goals is located in Appendix C. In this example, one area for peer review is successful identification and implementation of best practices to reduce hospital infection rates.

### Case Study—Decreasing VAP Using Peer Review

The awareness of evidence-based nursing measures for the prevention of ventilator-associated pneumonia (VAP) became widespread as the result of the Institute for Healthcare Improvement's 100,000 Lives Campaign in 2005. The aim of the initiative is to prevent patient mortality and morbidity, reduce the length of intensive care unit (ICU) and post-ICU hospital stays, and reduce overall costs (Institute for Healthcare Improvement, 2007). Participating organizations in this campaign that implemented the recommendations named the VAP bundle demonstrated significant success, many eliminating VAP in their organizations. Physicians, respiratory therapists, pharmacists, and nurses all play a unique role in the implementation of the VAP bundle. As a result of the impressive focused improvements in decreasing VAP, organizations that did not originally participate, created safety goals and processes to achieve similar results.

The first step in making this change involves the hospital's Quality Council setting a goal to decrease their overall VAP rates. The CNO provides leadership to this initiative by ensuring that this organizational VAP goal is incorporated into the nursing strategic plan and is assigned to the nursing shared governance leadership to define the nursing specific accountabilities and resources necessary to achieve this goal. Typically, it is the Nursing Evidence-Based Practice Council that endorses the following evidence-based interventions as standards of practice for all nurses caring for patients receiving ventilator support, as a result of their participation on an interdisciplinary VAP team:

- Elevation of the head of the bed (HOB) to between 30 and 45 degrees and oral care;
- Daily "sedative interruption" and daily assessment of readiness to extubate;
- Administration of peptic ulcer disease (PUD) prophylaxis; and
- Implementation of deep venous thrombosis (DVT) prophylaxis, unless contraindicated. (Evans, 2005)

After the Nursing Evidence-Based Practice Council's decision on the nursing VAP standards and protocol, the Nursing Quality and Safety Council creates the tools and processes to ensure the measurement of the interventions and outcomes to report at the hospital, unit, and provider levels. A sample of a peer-to-peer handoff tool used to monitor the first practice standard, involving elevating the HOB and oral care, is illustrated in Figure 5-3. There is an expectation that corrective action by the direct care practitioner is performed as soon as the deviation from the defined standards is identified. Education about this change, coordinated with the Nursing Professional Development Council, is an essential step in the readiness process.

The individual unit-based Nursing Quality/Peer Review Council reviews this data at regular intervals at their meetings. Hospital, unit, and blinded individual results are shared openly with council members using a report card format.

**Figure 5-3.   VAP QA monitoring tool.**

| VAP Nursing Quality Improvement—ICU/CCU/SNICU | | | | | |
|---|---|---|---|---|---|
| | BED 1 | | BED 2 | | BED 3 | |
| Oral Care Standards | YES | *NO | YES | *NO | YES | *NO |
| HOB elevated at least 30° | | | | | | |
| Teeth brushed this shift? | | | | | | |
| Peridex used? | | | | | | |
| Initials of Nurse reporting off _____ Date _____ Time _____ | | | | | | |
| *If "No"—describe corrective action taken: | | | | | | |
| Return to your unit's VAP QA box at the end of the shift. | | | | | | |

Nurses receive their individual report card from a member of the unit-based Nursing Quality/Peer Review Council along with recognition and praise for good performance when indicated.

Similar contributions of nursing in other organizations has helped decrease the rate of VAP to zero in many hospitals. Real-time feedback opportunities for performance enhancement using shift-to-shift peer review naturally occurs during patient handoffs and rounding. Targeting peer review processes simultaneous with actual care delivery as illustrated in this best practice leads to daily accountability for system wide outcomes management.

This practice incorporated the following peer review principles:

1.  *The peer is someone of the same rank.* In this case, it was direct care nurse to direct care nurse.
2.  *Peer review is practice focused.* The peer-to-peer feedback focused on VAP protocol standards as defined the Nursing Evidence-Based Practice Council.
3.  *Feedback is timely, routine, and a continuous expectation.* All nurses were engaged in achieving this goal and peer-to-peer feedback was scheduled at the time of the patient handoff. Any nurse observing deviations from the protocol was obligated to correct and report. Confidentiality of individual results was maintained by blinding the scorecards to others but reporting the outcomes to the Quality Council.
4.  *Peer review fosters a continuous learning culture of patient safety and best practice.* This project involved nurses from several councils

focusing on evidence-based practice in the development of the nursing protocol, creation of the monitoring process and tool, and subsequent education on the protocol. Frequent discussions of the results fostered continuous learning and engagement on patient safety.

5. *Feedback is not anonymous.* Peer-to-peer feedback was done face-to-face at the time of the handoff.

### Peer Review for Unit-Specific Safety Issues

The commonly collected and reported nurse-sensitive indicators such as falls, pressure ulcers, and urinary tract infections are not always pertinent in all practice areas. Some quality and safety initiatives are specialty specific and based on national nursing standards as is the case in following example from a perinatal nursing unit.

Direct care nurses on one perinatal unit were concerned about infant airway safety. The mother and baby nurses unit frequently identified that the bulb syringe for emergency clearing of the infant's airway was routinely missing from the infant's crib after transfer from the birthing center. It is a safety standard to have a bulb syringe at the bedside of each newborn throughout hospitalization. The mother/baby nurses expressed their concern to their unit-based Nursing Practice Council representatives. The Perinatal Practice Council recommended an educational approach to increase awareness of both the staff and patients for this safety standard followed by periodic monitoring. Several Practice Council members created a "Plant Your Bulb" awareness campaign. Informational posters were created for staff and families and placed throughout the unit in public places. Stickers were made and placed in the cribs showing where the bulb should be planted or located.

Compliance with this practice was measured using periodic real-time or impromptu spot checks of every occupied newborn crib on the unit. Direct care nurses performed these impromptu checks at different times and shifts throughout the specified monitoring period. If no bulb syringe was found during the spot check, immediate corrective action was taken to replace it. A review of data collection sheets, which follows in Table 5-2, revealed that the bulb syringe was often missing with new cesarean section births. Dialogue between the mother and baby nurses and birthing center nurses found that the bulb syringes used at delivery were often grossly contaminated with blood and thrown away without replacement of a fresh one in the operating room. Communication with the birthing center nurses about this safety concern and heightened surveillance from the mother and baby staff helped ensure the presence of a bulb syringe at each newborn's bedside. Staff expressed a positive response to this "no blame" approach to ensure patient safety.

**Table 5-2.   Perinatal QA Monitoring Sheet**

**Perinatal "Plant Your Bulb" Safety Audit**
**Please return to Shared Governance Mailbox when complete**

| Date: / /08 Room Number | Bulb in Crib | | Corrective Actions or Comments |
| --- | --- | --- | --- |
| | Yes | No | |
| 4401 | X | | |
| 4402 | | X | New C-Section—bulb syringe replaced |
| 4403 | X | | |
| 4404 | X | | |
| 4405 | X | | |
| 4406 | X | | |
| 4407 | X | | |
| 4408 | X | | |
| 4409 | | X | New C-Section—bulb syringe replaced |
| 4410 | X | | |
| 4411 | X | | |
| 4412 | X | | |
| 4413 | X | | |

This unit-based practice incorporated the following principles of peer review:

1. *The peer is someone of the same rank.* This process was created and monitored by direct care givers using their shared governance structure.
2. *Peer review is practice focused.* The peer-to-peer feedback focused on the national nursing standard for ensuring the infant's bulb syringe was readily available in the crib.
3. *Feedback is timely, routine, and a continuous expectation.* The impromptu spot checks engaged all direct care providers and increased awareness among the collective without fear of reprisal. Immediate corrective action, when warranted, helped ensure significant progress toward 100% compliance.
4. *Peer review fosters a continuous learning culture of patient safety and best practice.* An awareness campaign was used by the nurses to

communicate the continuous expectation around infant safety. The use of posters and stickers created by the nurses was creative and engaging for staff and patients

5. *Feedback is not anonymous.* The monitoring exercise focused on identifying and correcting deviations from the standard of care. Face-to-face dialogue among direct care providers from the two units helped to find the root cause and create heightened awareness that was sustainable.

## Individualizing Patient Specific Practice—TIPS

The most effective nursing interventions are individualized to the patient and family. The same is true for safety-focused initiatives as recognized by TJC in their patient safety standard that encourages patient's active involvement in their own plan of care, including safety strategies (TJC, 2008). This recommendation is based on the notion that when patients know what to expect, they are more aware of and can help alleviate safety hazards.

Targeting improvement for patient safety or TIPS is a simple process focused at achieving unit-focused quality and safety outcomes by individualizing care with the patient and family. The TIPS process further refines unit-based, point-of-service efforts to improve patient safety one day at a time. Focusing on simple and routine processes such as the handoff, helps hardwire nurse sensitive indicators into the nursing process (Harrington, 2009). As with other quality and safety initiatives, the unit-based shared governance councils provide leadership for these initiatives. The review of quality data by the unit's Nursing Quality/Peer Review council identifies targets for improvement for their specific populations. Next, the unit-based Practice Council designs evidence-based solutions to the specific patient care problems and implements these solutions through day-to-day, shift-to-shift communication using TIPS.

TIPS facilitates both peer-to-peer communication and improvements in patient care. Making TIPS part of the patient handoff creates a learning environment that heightens awareness of the unit's quality and safety initiatives while improving individual and collective outcomes through learning and collaboration. It is expected that, on a daily basis, all nurses communicate about the TIPS for the day. This creates the expectation that each caregiver knows about, is able to articulate, and acts upon the focus and results of their quality improvement activities.

TIPS also helps bring awareness to groups of nurses that are not always in the communication loop such as those who work part-time, per diem, or who have a floating assignment. TIPS allows staff to achieve great practice outcomes day after day through staff helping staff. It is essential that the Quality/Peer Review Council provide feedback about the results of these efforts on a regular basis.

## Using TIPS to Enhance Patient Satisfaction

Patient satisfaction is one example of a nurse-sensitive indicator that is reported collectively for the organization as well as at the individual unit level. It is common for the Nursing Quality and Safety Council to set annual benchmarks for patient satisfaction to improve patient satisfaction overall. Accordingly, each unit-based Quality/Peer Review Council identifies their patient satisfaction goals, benchmarks, and strategies to achieve the desired outcomes. Issues related to patient satisfaction vary from unit to unit and need to be modulated by direct care givers.

After review of their patient satisfaction data, the nurse representatives for the Quality/Peer Review Council on one busy surgical/orthopedic unit realized that call light response time was an area that needed improvement. They asked the unit-based Evidence Practice council to review best practices for enhancing satisfaction with call light response. Hourly rounding is one such practice and the unit subsequently designed and implemented focused hourly rounding. Nurses on this unit used TIPS for this focused quality and safety improvement as follows:

*T* – Target: The call light response time.

*I* – Improvement: The focus is to implement routine rounds that would help anticipate patient's needs and decrease the patient's need to use the call light. Hourly rounding included assessments for the most common reasons patient's use the call light: pain, potty, positioning, and possessions.

*P* – Patient: Nurses' individualized the plan of care related to the target with each patient. In one instance, a patient indicated pain control as their most important issue along with their desire to not be dependent on the nurses for this.

*S* – Safety: The patient's nurse developed an individualized plan of care for self-medication using evidenced-based practice and hospital safety rules. At the time of the patient handoff, during the TIPS of the day, this individualized plan of care was communicated to the next nurse along with expectations for evaluation of the plan and modifications as needed.

Several months after implementation of this approach to individualize the plan of care for each patient, the unit reported an increase in patient satisfaction related to call lights and also an increase in patient satisfaction related to pain management.

## TIPS to Decrease Falls on an Oncology Unit

In reviewing their most recent quality data, one oncology unit's Quality/Peer Review Council observed an increasing trend in the number of falls on their unit. They asked the unit-based Practice Council to review best practices for decreasing falls in this population. The council found that few studies have investigated specific risk factors from an oncology and palliative care perspective and concluded that more research was needed in this area. TIPS was used as a safety measure to individualize care using the evidence-based Hendrich II risk assessment tool for falls (already adopted for use in the organization). Prior to implementation, all staff participated in education on falls prevention that included the hospital falls prevention protocol and patient and family education awareness campaign. TIPS implementation for this focused quality and safety improvement was as follows:

*T –* Target: To decrease each patients risk for falling.

*I –* Improvement: Focus is for the oncology unit to be at or below the national benchmark for falls by using the risk assessment tool.

*P –* Patients: Patients and families were educated about the falls prevention program, including specific interventions related to their fall risk assessment. One patient opposed having to waiting for assistance to get up and stated, "I am not sick. I am only here for chemotherapy therefore should be able to get to bathroom alone."

*S –* Safety: In partnership with the patient and family, the nurse developed an individualized plan of care, identifying hourly rounds on this patient and agreement from the patient that he will anticipate assistance on an hourly basis. At the time of the patient handoff, during the TIPS of the day, this individualized plan of care was communicated to the next nurse along with expectations for evaluation of the plan and modification as needed. The result of the focused unit-based actions kept these patients free of falls, whereas the unit-based council designed a research proposal to address the needs of their specific patient population.

TIPS incorporates the following principles of peer review:

1. *The peer is someone of the same rank.* Direct care nurses identified their unit's Targeted Improvement for Patient Safety and communicated this directly to each other at the time of the patient handoff along with individualized patient care plans related to the target.

2. *Peer review is practice focused.* The peer-to-peer feedback focused on ensuring the safety focus off of the unit and utilized evidence-based practice protocols where appropriate.

3. *Feedback is timely, routine, and a continuous expectation.* TIPS is designed to be a continuous awareness of the patient safety issues that are of the highest concern in a patient care area. TIPS incorporates evidence-based practices into individualized focused safety efforts and is designed to achieve rapid results.

4. *Peer review fosters a continuous learning culture of patient safety and best practice.* The use of posters, e-mails, face-to-face handoffs,

and patient and family education was a dynamic process on both of the busy acute care areas.

5. *Feedback is not anonymous.* Daily face-to-face dialogue on TIPS among direct care providers engages direct care providers in collective efforts toward enhancing patient safety.

**Summary of Peer Review for Quality and Safety**

The Nursing Quality and Safety Council provides the direction and oversight for achieving of quality care through a continuous peer review program. Daily peer review is the professional practice process that ensures that outcomes are achieved. The unit-based councils, using evidence-based practices and the peer review process, plan, develop, execute, and evaluate the care of each patient individually. TIPS allows for the autonomy of the practitioner at the bedside to develop an individualized plan for each patient and to utilize his or her critical thinking skills to engage with the patient and family to identify a process of improvement that works for and with them. TIPS also provides a daily focus on quality that enhances communication among all members of the team.


**PEER REVIEW FOCUS ON ROLE ACTUALIZATION**

As knowledge workers, nurses use evidence-based practices to drive the outcomes of their work. Continually amending and extending both nursing knowledge and skills promotes organizational effectiveness as well as organizational survival. Peer review plays an essential role in promoting continued learning, nursing role and practice development, and nursing role autonomy. In the *Guide to the Code of Ethics for Nurses: Interpretation and Application* (ANA, 2008), the concept of professional growth moves beyond minimal standards of nursing, often referred to as competencies, toward an ideal of excellence in practice. It goes on to define a shift in emphasis on professional growth from the duty to self to a duty to the profession and for the sake of the profession.

Peer-to-peer feedback is an expected behavior throughout orientation and socialization to new roles. Once formal orientation is completed, however, most cultures abandon the expectation of daily feedback around one's practice, to the detriment of the profession and organization. The adult education literature informs that feedback promotes learning and that expanding capacity for self-direction and self-assessment requires practice with feedback and cannot be assumed by virtue of age (Fiddler, Marienau, & Whitaker, 2006) or years of experience. Therefore, it is essential to extend this fundamental practice of giving and receiving peer-to-peer feedback beyond orientation to achieve continuous clinical practice development along the beginner-to-expert framework throughout one's career.

Protecting nurse's role autonomy and the stature of nursing as a profession requires peer review to foster professional development as well as to ensure role competency. Although widely used to define proficiency, the ANA defines competence as being the rock bottom level of acceptable practice and the level below, which no practitioner should fall (ANA, 2008). Therefore, is it time to move away from the minimalist concept of competency and to utilize peer review for professional credentialing and privileging.

## Structure and Alignment for Nursing Professional Development

The Nursing Professional Development Council and the APN Council, as applicable, have primary responsibility for setting goals related to professional development for direct care nurses, nurse educators, and APNs. The involvement of both of these councils in peer review is substantial in evaluating and measuring the quality of nursing education and nursing educators; nursing competency, credentialing, and privileging; and professional advancement processes and procedures. The Nursing Professional Development Council is responsible for ensuring that educational needs of all levels of nurses in the organization are directed at maintaining competency and supporting continuous professional development to ensure quality and safety outcomes. This council directs and coordinates nursing orientation, nurse residency programs, experienced nurse's professional development, and professional advancement processes and procedures. This includes developing and monitoring all clinical ladder and clinical advancement programs for the nursing. Concepts of learning environments and the evidence-based novice-to-expert practitioner theories should be integrated into the advancement processes. When an APN council is active, all aspects of APN professional development and peer review will be located within the APN Council.

It is important to identify expectations for practice behaviors at different development stages of nurses as a "nurse is not a nurse is not a nurse." The ANA 1988 peer review guidelines identified this important point and gave guidance accordingly in the statement that "the Peer reviewers are nurse colleagues with clinical competence similar to that of the nurse seeking peer review" (p. 5). Decades of research by Dr. Patricia Benner and others defines the wide range of practice distinctions of nurses from different backgrounds and experiences. Expectations of practice at each level must be understood as illustrated by Drs. Patricia and Richard Benner in the following statements:

> Because developing clinical expertise is based on experiential learning, the practitioner at each stage . . . can be the best practitioner at whatever stage of the model (novice to expert)—best beginning practitioner, the best possible

competent level practitioner, and at the proficient and expert stages, be astute at recognizing the unexpected subtle deviations from normal . . . What is not possible or reasonable is to expect clinicians to practice beyond their own experience level with any particular patient population. This is an obvious statement but is often ignored in a technical vision or practice, where it is imagined that critical pathways and protocols can make explicit the myriad trajectories and variations in practice. Nevertheless, clinicians cannot be held accountable for what they have not had the opportunity to learn in their practice. But they can work in a collaborative climate where the collective goal is to make the best use of the experiential wisdom of one's colleagues and all experiential learning. (Haag-Heitman, 1999, p. 27)

Rich opportunities exist for role actualization using peer review to be guided by the Nursing Professional Development Council. These include nursing orientation, preceptor training, nurse residency programs, clinical advancement, competency validation, and nurse educator, and direct care nurses privileging and credentialing.

## Advancing the Practice of Nurse Educators Using Peer Review

If a department of nursing education or unit-based educators exists in the organization, then a component of practice advancement is indicated for these practitioners. The process of peer review for the educators includes the evaluation of teaching techniques and methods, effectiveness as rated by the learners, and the quantity of classes taught. Standards for educator performance that can be used for peer review evolve from national standards for nurse educators as defined by the National League for Nursing and the National Nursing Staff Development Organization. Organizational specific expectations should also be incorporated in peer review.

Educator peer review processes include direct observation of teaching interactions by other educators using established criteria, review of formal class evaluations from learners, and the review of outcomes achieved from educational interventions. Educators are held accountable for development of new techniques for learning in the clinical setting using evidence-based education practices.

## Nursing Professional Role Actualization: Orientation, Preceptor Training, and Nurse Residency Programs

The Nursing Professional Development Council is responsible for ensuring the orientation of new graduate and experienced nurses is done using a process that is learner focused, systematic, and evidence based. There is mounting evidence for the necessity of extending the learning experience for new graduates into a formal guided nurse residency program. Ensuring the quality of the process and the quality of the trainers or preceptors for both orientation and the nurse residency programs is the work of the Nursing Professional Development Council.

Expectations for the nurse preceptor's role need to be standardized and explicit in the role description. All preceptors need specific training and competency validation for this role. Preceptors at or one stage above the developmental stage of the nurse in orientation best facilitates learning for the new hire. For example, new graduates are at the novice stage and preceptors at the advanced beginner stage are ideal as they understand these learners' unique issues and challenges. Accordingly, expert nurses need preceptors at the expert stage to assist in the on-boarding process of experienced nurses. Matching the developmental stage of the learner and the preceptor ensures that the developmental stage of the nurse is integrated into peer review.

Frequent feedback about the accomplishment of learner objectives, goals, and performance using the principles of peer review creates a supportive learning environment. Peer review should also be incorporated into the formal preceptor evaluation along with feedback about other aspects of the orientation. Preceptors should use this feedback to enhance their individual performance. Collective feedback about preceptors performance is used to enhance the orientation process overall and guide preceptor development.

These peer review practices incorporate the following principles of peer review:

1. *The peer is someone of the same rank.* Matching the developmental stage of the learner and preceptor ensures the developmental stage of the nurse at the same rank is integrated into peer review.
2. *Peer review is practice focused.* Utilizing principles from adult education and the novice-to-expert research makes this practice focused and evidence based.
3. *Feedback is timely, routine, and a continuous expectation.* Frequent feedback about the learner's objective is incorporated into the peer review. Preceptors also receive feedback to enhance their individual performance.
4. *Peer review fosters a continuous learning culture of patient safety and best practice.* Ensuring the quality of the process and quality of the trainers for both orientation and nurse residency programs fosters continuous learning.
5. *Feedback is not anonymous.* In all cases, feedback is not anonymous.
6. *Feedback incorporates the developmental stage of the nurse.* Utilizing the novice to expert framework identifies the expected characteristics of practice at stage to incorporate in feedback.

### Nursing Professional Development Council—Practice Advancement

Many organizations developed clinical and career ladder programs in the 1980s as popular adjuncts to recruitment and retention during the nursing shortage. These programs were used for recognition and differentiation of practice. There appears to be a resurgence of interest in these programs again during this current nursing shortage. Historically, these processes rarely used a true peer review process from nurses at the same level for review and determination of the applicant's advancement. Commonly, it is the manager who is the gatekeeper and final decision maker in this process. Typical criteria used in these programs includes continuing education credit, committee participation, work experience, certifications, academic degrees, community service, and performance appraisal scores (Schmidt, Nelson, & Godfrey, 2003) often involving elaborate portfolios. Although many programs claim to use Benner's (1984) work as an organizing framework, they lack a true correlation between the advancement criteria used in the clinical ladders and Benner's developmental criteria that is measured solely by exemplars from practice. Participation rates are typically low with nurses citing unrealistic expectations, time-consuming processes and inconsistencies in the program administration as the many deterrents.

Research into clinical practice development indicates that both personal and environmental factors influence the development along a novice-to-expert continuum as illustrated by Haag-Heitman (2008). Note, time and service do not equate to the movement along the development continuum and not all nurses will attain the expert stage of performance (see Figure 5-4).

An adjunct-to-clinical ladders, as just previously described, is the authentic peer review model based on the novice-to-expert model previously described in *Clinical Practice Development: Using Novice to Expert Theory* (Haag-Heitman,

---

**Figure 5-4.  Factors that influence clinical practice development.**

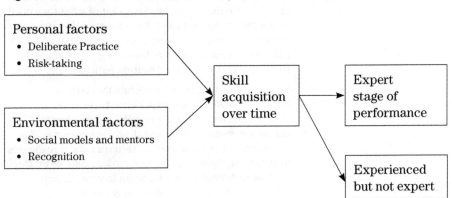

1999). Actual stories of a nurse's performance with patients and families, defined by their individual stories from practice, are the foundation for this advancement process. This approach acknowledges that essential nursing behaviors at each developmental stage are not always readily observable but are visible in individual narrative accounts of nursing practice. This clinical practice development advancement model is grounded in a beginner-to-expert framework, incorporating the domains of clinical knowledge and decision making, education of patient and family, professional development, coordination and collaboration, and caring (see Table 5-3). These domains of clinical practice for this model were drawn from the organization's nursing conceptual framework and nursing model of care. These domains of clinical practice became the framework for measuring the nurse's developmental stage.

**Table 5-3. Definitions of Stages of Clinical Practice Development**

| Stage | Definition |
|---|---|
| 1<br>Novice | The Stage 1 novice nurse is a new graduate of an RN program and is in orientation. This nurse is obtaining knowledge and experience in clinical and technical skills. Under the guidance of a preceptor, the nurse collects objective data according to guidelines and rules obtained from nursing education and in orientation. The novice nurse utilizes this objective data and seeks assistance in making clinical decisions. |
| 2<br>Advanced Beginner | Stage 2 advanced beginners are guided by policies, procedures, and standards. They are building a knowledge base through practice and are most comfortable in a task environment. They describe a clinical situation from the viewpoint of what they need to do, rather than relating the context of the situation or how the patient responds. Advanced beginners practice from a theoretical knowledge base while they recognize and provide for routine patient needs. |
| 3<br>Competent | Stage 3 competent nurses integrate theoretical knowledge with clinical experience in the care of patients and families. Care is delivered utilizing a deliberate, systematic approach and practice is guided by increasing awareness of patterns of patient responses in recurrent situations. The nurses demonstrate mastery of most technical skills, and begin to view clinical situations from a patient and family focus. |

| Stage | Definition |
|-------|-----------|
| 4<br>Proficient | Stage 4 nurses are proficient practitioners who have in-depth knowledge of nursing practice, perceive situations as a whole, and comprehend the significant elements based on previous experience. These nurses demonstrate the ability to recognize situational changes that require unplanned or unanticipated interventions. They respond to most situations with confidence, speed, and flexibility. Progression is from task orientation to a holistic view of patient care. The nurses develop effective relationships with other caregivers and provide leadership within the healthcare team to formulate integrated approaches to care. They interpret the patient and family experiences from a perspective that begins to envision and create possibilities. |
| 5<br>Expert | Stage 5 nurses are expert practitioners whose intuition and skill arise from comprehensive knowledge grounded in experience. Their practice is characterized by a flexible, innovative, and confident self-directed approach to patient and family care. Expert nurses operate from a deep understanding of the total situation. They put into perspective their own personal values and are able to encourage and support patient and family choices. Expert nurses collaborate with other caregivers to challenge and coordinate institutional resources to maximize advocacy for patient and family care in achieving the most effective outcomes. |

Source: From *Clinical Practice Development Using Novice to Expert Theory*, by B. Haag-Heitman, 1999, Gaithersburg, MD: Aspen. Copyright 1999 by Aspen. Reprinted with permission.

A clinical advancement design work group of mostly direct care nurses, commissioned by the Nursing Practice Council, developed this model. Prior to selecting the novice-to-expert model, the work group members identified the following important elements for successful implementation (Gray, 1999). The model should:

- Measure outcomes and be based on nursing behavioral language and practice;
- Not have the manager as "gatekeeper," but rather, as coach and mentor;
- Be comprehensive and universal across settings and continuum of care;
- Reflect mission, vision, and values;
- Be user-friendly, not cumbersome, and easily understood;
- Include links to research and outcome facilitation;

- Be flexible and can evolve with practice;
- Ensure opportunities for growth and mentorship;
- Provide a celebration of practice and recognition;
- Define growth behaviors along the continuum;
- Create a correlation between salary and advancement;
- Create a correlation between increased development and increased opportunity;
- Be applicable to nurses across practice settings;
- Adopt a novice-to-expert framework;
- Include participation of all staff;
- Include job descriptions that vary according to developmental stage; and
- Include writing two to three clinical narratives "exemplars" and presentation to peer review panel of expert staff nurses for advancement.

The peer review promotional advancement panel composition includes expert direct care nurses whose practice is described by the beginner-to-expert model and who themselves have participated in the advancement process. To become a peer review panel member, direct care nurses need to also demonstrate good interpersonal and group skills, professional commitment, knowledge, and the skill to assess and give constructive feedback related to the beginner-to-expert framework. The shared leadership training described in Chapter 6 helped develop panel members for this peer review role.

These peer review practices incorporate the following principles of peer review:

1. *The peer is someone of the same rank.* This model began to define that rank is more than just job title and includes the developmental continuum of novice to expert.
2. *Peer review is practice focused.* The novice-to-expert framework evolved from direct practice domains. Practice exemplars are used to enhance the stage of development.
3. *Feedback is timely, routine, and a continuous expectation.* The feedback was routine and continuous such as every nurse was part of the peer review process. Timelines were self-determined by the nurse as they applied for recognition of their practice development at the next stage.
4. *Peer review fosters a continuous learning culture of patient safety and best practice.* Shared leadership training helped develop panel members for the peer review role.
5. *Feedback is not anonymous.* Feedback was never anonymous and a peer-to-peer celebration was part of the recognition process.
6. *Feedback incorporates the developmental stage of the nurse.* Feedback focused solely or the developmental stage of the nurse.

**Peer Competency Validation: Challenging the Concept of Traditional "Skills Days"**

The Nursing Professional Development Council's role is to direct the unit-level councils to review and determine the educational needs and competencies of the staff related to their unique patients' populations. To facilitate this work, the unit-based councils should annually identify new patient populations and new technology that need competency validation. In addition, the Nursing Professional Development Council reviews their unit-based critical incidents to recognize patterns in knowledge and skill deficits that are impeding quality and safety.

As with other processes, much of the work related to nursing clinical competency assessment has been directed by management and educators using annual "skills day." Considerable resources are invested in these skills days annually that usually entail the repetitive process of nurses going from station to station to demonstrate a clinical skill in a static environment. This process lacks true correlation between performance in this environment and actual performance in a clinical situation as many times the performance deficits are coached to ensure passing of the competency. Case in point, usually no one flunks CPR in the classroom.

Some organizations are beginning to utilize new approaches, using peers to define the competencies needed and validate performance in real time in actual situations. This shift incorporates the following principles:

- Moving from traditional psychomotor to interpersonal and critical thinking domains;
- Discovering the most accurate way of assessing competency at the point of care and bedside; and
- Recognizing the peers as an essential source of learning.

The following examples illustrate one organization's process and enhanced research-based outcomes from moving from a traditional approach to peer review competency validation model of one organization (Ringerman, Flint, & Hughes, 2006). These authors started by doing a force field analysis, one of the primary tools in quality management (Figure 5-5).

The outcomes of this best practice included:

1. Reduction in number of competencies from the traditional 12 to 3 to 5
2. Increase in rationale for competency selection
3. Implementation of interraterreliability
4. Assurance that 100% of staff was validated in the specified time frame
5. Staff satisfaction with the process
   a. "much better than the old process"
   b. "more effective"

**Figure 5-5.    Force field analysis for peer competency model.**

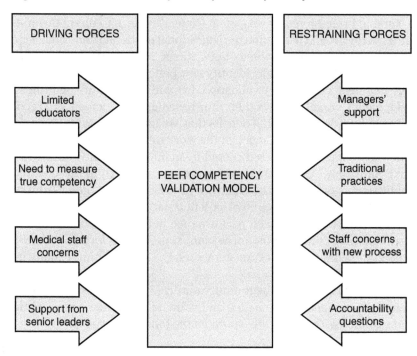

c. "creates accountability"
d. no negatives
6. Decreased Cost
   a. $28,477 savings over 1 year (for four departments)
   b. exceeded goal of being budget neutral (Ringerman *et al.*, 2006)

These peer review practices incorporate the following principles of peer review:

1. *The peer is someone of the same rank.* The direct care nurses were validated to measure competency.
2. *Peer review is practice focused.* The competencies were practiced focused.
3. *Feedback is timely, routine, and a continuous expectation.* Feedback was given in real time during competency assessed by the peer.
4. *Peer review fosters a continuous learning culture of patient safety and best practice.* There were 30% of staff not validated on the first attempt leading to individualized learning plans. The three domains of

psychomotor, interpersonal interaction, and critical thinking were consistently applied for all identified competencies.
5. *Feedback is not anonymous.* Feedback was done peer-to-peer, face-to-face.

Another best practice example of competency validation from Decatur Memorial Hospital, Decatur, Illinois is located in Appendix D.

## Nursing Professional Role Actualization: Privileging and Credentialing

Each state's Nurse Practice Act addresses the accountability and authority of nursing roles and peer review processes as applicable. Most states do not have mandated reporting for nursing peer review; however, several states such as Texas and New Jersey do require reporting in certain situations. To help illustrate the differences between mandatory state reporting and hospital quality and safety improvement efforts, information about the Texas Board of Nursing Peer Review is located in Appendix E. Every nurse needs to be familiar with their state's nursing practice act. Beyond licensing and other legal regulations, a well-developed and rigorous credentialing and privileging process is essential for building a quality professional staff.

In a shared governance framework, staff must have accountability for appropriate credentialing of applicants to the nursing staff as the exercise of the clinical nurse role is a privilege, and not an obligation (Porter-O'Grady, 1985). In clinical roles, the majority of credentials are clinical and this demands that the clinical staff play a significant role in review of their peers' credentials. The same applies to nurses in educator, management, and advanced practice roles. Ensuring the appropriate preparation of clinical roles to meet the specified needs of patients is a function of the Nursing Professional Development Council. Role privileging incorporates academic preparation, degrees, appropriate licensure, certifications, previous experiences, and other documents indicating adequate preparation. The shared governance bylaws should define the credentialing and privileging processes for nursing.

In the case of APNs or other nurses seeking privileges on the hospital staff, the bylaws should indicate these nurses first pass the nursing credentials review (Porter-O'Grady, 1985). An example of APN credentialing is included in the APN council section later in this chapter. Best practices for direct care nurse credentialing and privileging that is an area that needs development.

## Summary of Peer Review for Role Actualization

The Nursing Professional Development Council provides direction and oversight for role actualization and peer review. Peer review plays an important role in ensuring that quality educational processes are in place to promote quality care providers. The Nursing Professional Development Council must define the peer review processes used to guarantee quality nursing orientation, preceptor training, nurse residency programs, clinical advancement, competency validation, and privileging and credentialing for nursing roles.

## PEER REVIEW FOCUS ON ADVANCING THE PRACTICE

### Structure and Alignment

The Nursing Evidence-Based Practice Council is responsible for advancing the practice of nursing with evidenced-based practice and research. This council addresses issues related to the standards of practice and the model of care. Peer review plays a critical role in ensuring adherence to these standards and the model of care, as well as identifying barriers or gaps in practice that need to be addressed.

Several examples are provided that illustrate the essential role of peer review in advancing practice. The first focus is on moving from traditional to evidence-based breastfeeding practices. The second involves the application of an evidence-based implementation of incident-based peer reviews for nursing, fashioned after the medical staff model of peer review involving formal case peer review. The third example is the use of evidence-based practice in the Post Anesthesia Care Unit. An innovative example that is not directly focused on patient care issues is the use of an internal peer review process to help ensure abstracts, posters, and podium presentations disseminated for external presentation represent the best scholarship. This innovative practice, courtesy of the Porter Adventist Hospital Evidence-Based Practice Council, is described more fully in Appendix F.

### Using Peer Review to Advance Practice: Using EBP

Achieving excellence in quality outcomes often involves implementing new practice standards and leaving traditional approaches to care behind. Abolishing time honored care approaches requires a well-defined plan, education, peer feedback, and leadership to ensure success. The following case study illustrates the essential role of peer review in moving from traditional care practices to evidenced-based care approaches.

Achieving international breastfeeding quality standards and outcomes using nursing's support of breastfeeding mothers requires integrating foundational science along with each individual mother's unique circumstances. The complexity of nursing care and support for breastfeeding is frequently discounted by those outside the specialty because of the perception that breastfeeding is a "natural" bodily function. However, new mothers often report receiving

**Table 5-4.  Baby Friendly Breastfeeding Standards**

**Ten Steps to Successful Breastfeeding for Hospitals**

1. Maintain a written breastfeeding policy that is routinely communicated to all healthcare staff.
2. Train all healthcare staff in skills necessary to implement this policy.
3. Inform all pregnant women about the benefits and management of breastfeeding.
4. Help mother initiate breastfeeding within 1 hour of birth.
5. Show mothers how to breastfeed and how to maintain lactation, even if they are separated from their infants.
6. Give infants no food or drink other that breastmilk, unless medically indicated.
7. Practice "rooming in"—allow mothers and infants to remain together 24 hours a day.
8. Encourage unrestricted breastfeeding.
9. Give no pacifiers or artificial nipples to breastfeeding infants.
10. Foster the establishment of breastfeeding support groups and refer mother to them on discharge from the hospital or clinic.

Source: From "The Ten Steps To Successful Breastfeeding," by BFHI USA, 2010, http://www.babyfriendlyusa.org/eng/10steps.html. Copyright 2010 by BFUSA. Reprinted with permission.

conflicting information and guidance about breastfeeding from nursing staff as well as from their family and friends. This inconsistency often leads to confusion, self-doubt, and a dissatisfactory experience, leading to early discontinuing of breastfeeding for some mothers. Achieving consistent nursing approaches to support breastfeeding is complicated by traditional nursing and folk practices surrounding breastfeeding during the postpartum period and first few months of life.

To address these issues and to strive to provide the highest quality of care possible, one hospital in this case study chose to adopt the practice standards defined by the Baby Friendly Hospital Initiative of the World Health Organization/United Nations Children's Fund (BFHI USA, 2010). As a first step in the planning phase, the unit-based Nursing Practice Council endorsed the Ten Steps to Successful Breastfeeding for Hospitals and agreed to adopt their practice standards as seen in Table 5-4.

A multidisciplinary steering committee of interested staff, certified lactation consultants, APNs, and nursing supervisors formed to guide the process and report back to the unit-based Practice Council on progress and practice change recommendations. The steering committee's role included:

- Performance of gap analysis for each step
- Recommending practice changes to the unit-based practice council
- Periodic measurement toward achieving the standards

- Communication with staff, physicians, and midwives
- Education of staff, physicians, and midwives
- Coordination and participation with the Baby Friendly application and on-site appraisal visit

Each of the ten steps has well-defined criteria and performance standards. The nursing staff enthusiastically united about this initiative. Initially, the Nursing Practice Council adopted the following approaches to bring about this practice changes:

- Group education,
- Updates and announcements at staff meetings,
- Computerized training,
- Articles with post tests,
- Posters, and
- Written reminders for staff not following the criteria.

Some changes in practices were easier to change than others. Staff achieved early success in implementing the written policy in the first step and initiating breastfeeding within an hour of birth for the fourth step. Several other steps proved more difficult and, despite many laborious efforts, the adherence to the standards proved inconsistent. Feeling very frustrated, the staff-led Baby Friendly committee requested managerial support to speak to noncompliant staff. Staff expressed fear and hesitancy to speak with their peers directly and some held the belief that feedback was a managerial duty under their union contract. The manager used the principles from the ANA *Guidelines for Peer Review* (1988) to assist in clarifying the role of staff-to-staff feedback and peer review about practice issues. The unit-based Quality Council helped the staff identify new strategies, including real-time audits of current patients on the units and using face-to-face practice-based dialogue about the new practice standards with their peers. To prepare staff for these types of person-to-person practice-focused interactions, mandatory sessions on giving and receiving feedback for all staff were held at the recommendation of the unit-based Practice Council with guidance from the Department of Organizational Development.

The staff of the Baby Friendly committee conducted the audits with the nursing staff during the shift-to-shift report. Nurses from both shifts meet together in the conference room for patient report, creating a natural group setting for team learning. One of most challenging of the 10 standards was the sixth, "Give infants no food or drink other than breastmilk, unless medically indicated" (BFHI USA, 2010). This was a dramatic departure from the traditional nursing practice of liberally feeding formula to breastfeeding babies to promote night-time sleep for the new mother, or attempting to satisfy unidentifiable infant cues that *possibly* indicated hunger. As each nurse reported off, he or she was asked if any of the breastfeeding infants in their care were supplemented during their shift. If yes, the Baby Friendly representative inquired about the medical indications for the supplementation. If medical indications existed, the Baby Friendly representative gave positive feedback and helped ensure documentation of the required elements. When no medical indication was evident, the Baby Friendly committee member reviewed the criteria for supplementation with the nurse, reinforced the practice standards, and discussed alternative to care. During these interactions, additional questions regarding breastfeeding issues and dilemmas arose and care strategies were offered, all which further advanced the practice. The real-time audit strategy enhanced compliance with the new standards and further enhanced breastfeeding knowledge of all staff. The Advanced Practice Registered Nurses supported the staff and helped facilitate the real-time audits. To prevent concerns about punitive or disciplinary actions, the process excluded management participation.

Step nine, "Give no pacifiers or artificial nipples to breastfeeding infants" (BFHI USA, 2010), also proved challenging. The Baby Friendly committee used the same face-to-face, real-time audit strategy. They also created a poster of the real-time audit results to help educate, show improvements, and reinforce this step. As illustrated in Figure 5-6, for each audit date, the placement of smiley faces on the chart indicated meeting the standard, and frowning faces indicated the criteria was not met. This feedback illustrates a nonpunitive, creative way to communicate expectations and findings. This peer-to-peer review helped meet the practice standard, was inexpensive, educational in nature, and overall was effective in advancing the practice. Notice that it took place outside any formal performance appraisal program or management interaction.

Baby Friendly Step #9

Give No Pacifiers or Artificial Nipples to Breastfeeding Infants
Each day a real-time audit was done to see if our breastfeed babies had pacifiers.
Each box with a face represents a breastfeeding baby.
If the baby had no pacifier, it was indicated by a smiley face on the chart ☺.
When a pacifier was found in the bed, or in a baby's mouth, it was indicated by a sad face ☹.

## Using Peer Review to Advance Practice: Incident-Based Peer Review

This form of nursing peer review is based on actual or "near miss" adverse events or occurrences. When a referral is made to the Evidence-Based Practice Council for case review, the referral is confidential and functions in accordance with the requirements of the State Nurse Practice Act and the bylaws of the Nursing Division. Members who participate in the review should have extensive protection against incurring civil liability during this section of the Evidence-Based Practice Council discussion.

**Figure 5-6.    Baby-friendly audit tool.**

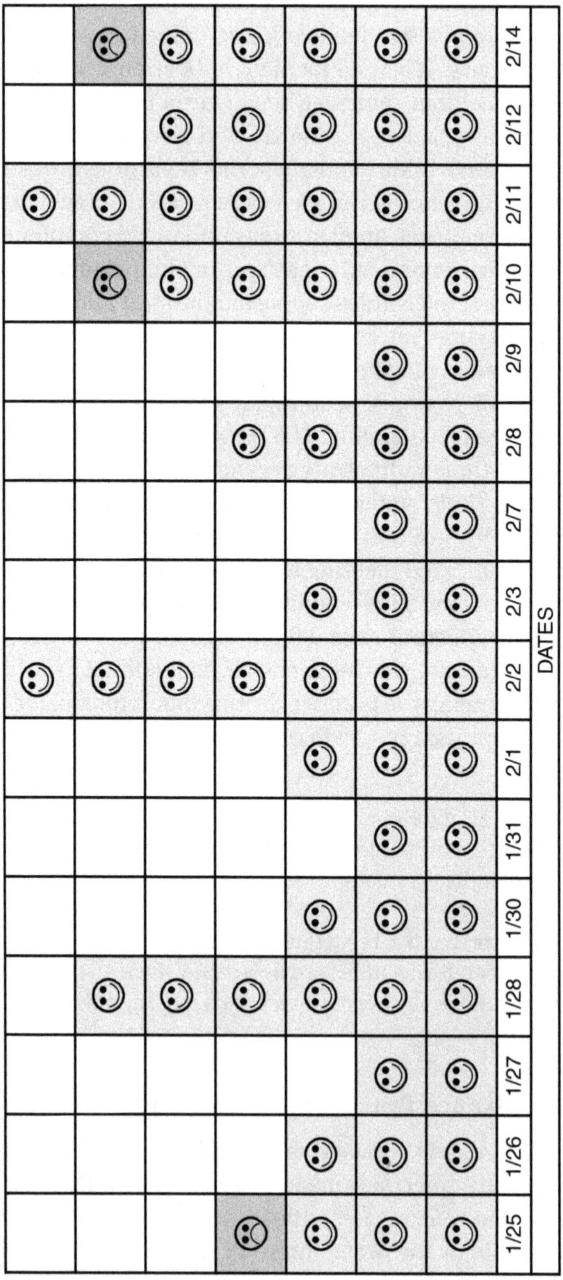

| | 1/25 | 1/26 | 1/27 | 1/28 | 1/30 | 1/31 | 2/1 | 2/2 | 2/3 | 2/7 | 2/8 | 2/9 | 2/10 | 2/11 | 2/12 | 2/14 |
|---|---|---|---|---|---|---|---|---|---|---|---|---|---|---|---|---|
| | ☺ | ☺ | ☺ | ☺ | ☺ | ☺ | ☺ | ☺ | ☺ | ☺ | ☺ | ☺ | ☺ | ☺ | ☺ | ☺ |
| | ☺ | ☺ | ☺ | ☺ | ☺ | ☺ | ☺ | ☺ | ☺ | ☺ | ☺ | ☺ | ☺ | ☺ | ☺ | ☺ |
| | ☺ | ☺ | | ☺ | ☺ | | | ☺ | | | ☺ | | ☺ | ☺ | | ☺ |
| | ☹ | | | ☺ | | | | ☺ | | | | | ☹ | ☺ | | ☹ |
| | | | | ☺ | | | | ☺ | | | | | | ☺ | | |
| | | | | | | | | ☺ | | | | | | ☺ | | |

DATES

SUNY Downstate Medical Center developed case review as part of their peer review process and identified common occurrences that lead to referrals as listed

- Events involving wrong patient, wrong procedure, wrong site
- Error of omission leading to death or serious injury
- Failure to rescue leading to significant deterioration of patient's condition
- Medication error with actual or potential serious harm, near death, or death
- Falls with fracture or head injury
- Any patient care situation that jeopardizes patient safety

A case study illustrating a medication error that had potential for harm is presented in the description of the development of their peer review process, provided in Appendix G.

OSF Rockford Hospital in Rockford, Illinois, a Magnet organization, also implemented nursing peer case review. They identify that referral sources and potential outcomes for case reviews. Referral sources can include:

- Risk/quality/performance improvement data,
- Nursing managements referral,
- Nursing peer referral,
- Physician/other providers referral,
- Pharmacy error, or
- Patient relations complaints.

Council decisions, post case review, might include:

- Nurse self-acknowledged action plan sufficient
- Educational offering
- Individual counseling and discussion
- Formulation of new policy or procedure.
- System opportunity: Refer to Quality Patient Safety Council
- Medical staff opportunity: Refer to medical staff
- Refer to nursing manager for formal corrective action, such as department manager developing a formal improvement plan with monitoring
- Nursing practice standards issue; Forward to nursing manager

*Case Study*: Review of this case focuses on safety concerns related to perioperative temperature management related to oversedation of an elderly patient that led to life-sustaining intervention to prevent complications. A 70-year-old woman was admitted for hip surgery following a fall in her home. She was very anxious about the surgery, and stated that she was recently widowed and fearful that she would never be able to care for herself or return to her home following recovery. Her vital signs were stable upon admission with the exception of being hypothermic at 96.4°F. The patient stated she was always cold, and ran a low temperature, which was normal for her. The RN working in the surgical holding area administered the preoperative IV sedation according to both the physician's order and the nursing procedure. Another dose of sedation followed shortly after, as the first dose did not have the desired effect. Shortly after, the patient became somnolent and was barely responsive. Severe respiratory depression followed and the patient required resuscitation.

Upon review of the nursing documentation, it was noted that the nurse had followed hospital and nursing protocols for sedation. Review of the nursing protocol indicated that it lacked hypothermia as a risk factor and did not reflect evidence-based practice. It was determined that this was a system problem and a new, evidence-based protocol was needed. The Evidence-Based Practice Council developed a new protocol using the ASPAN Clinical Guidelines (2002), and referred to the Professional Development Council to define and implement an education plan for all direct care providers.

A full description of the policy and procedure used at OSF Rockford in Rockford, Illinois, a Magnet organization, for implementation of critical incident debriefing is provided in Appendix H.

**Advancing Nursing Practice: Implementing Open Visitation in the PACU**

Concepts of open visitation have been firmly grounded in the nursing research for the past 25 years. The American Society of PeriAnesthesia Nurses (ASPAN) Position Statement on Visitation in Phase 1 Level of Care (2007) was first proposed in 2003. Historically, Post Anesthesia Care Units (PACU) have been not routinely permitted family members to visit or participate in the care of their family member. A patient's family waited anxiously while the patient recovered in the PACU. In recent years there have been rapid advances in anesthesia management with shorter acting anesthetic agents and increased use of regional anesthetic techniques. There is a growing body of evidence in support of visitation and support presence at the bedside. ASPAN supports the reevaluation of the needs of both patients and families while striving to maintain quality services across the continuum of patient care. In response to concerns of many Perianesthesia nurses from around the country, the Standards and Guidelines Committee conducted a review of literature and gathered information from various institutions in order to identify issues related to visitation in Phase I level of care. (ASPAN, 2007)

One organization was successful in the implementation of this new standard as decided by the unit-based Practice Council in the PACU. The Practice Council chair returned from the ASPAN conference with the position statement on visitation as a new evidence-based practice standard. Upon review, the Practice Council recognized the need for practice change, adopted the guidelines from the ASPAN position, and began working on an implementation plan. To facilitate this change, the Practice Council required each nurse review the position statement for the proposed practice change. Initially, some nurses were dissatisfied with the practice change, but through education and continuous peer review, nursing satisfaction and engagement increased. Patients and families commented on their positive satisfaction with the practice change, similar to those in the position statement, such as "not being treated as visitors with restricted access, but active participates in their family's care" (ASPAN, 2003). The annual report to the Board of Trustees included the accomplishments of this goal.

### Summary of Peer Review for Advancing the Practice

The Nursing Evidence-Based Practice Council defines the practice of nursing based on evidenced-based practice and research. Peer review plays a major role in implementing practice changes and overcoming traditional approaches to care. In addition to helping ensure adherence to practice standards, peer review can also play a role in the evaluation of the model of care. By the development of job descriptions, standards of performance, career ladders, and novice expert models, the shared governance councils begin to hardwire the concepts outlined in the model of care into these documents. In so doing, these documents become a frame of reference for all practitioners and can be used in peer review.

### APN PEER REVIEW

Peer review of Advanced Practice Registered Nurses' (APRNs) practice is essential but often neglected in organizations. APRNs include clinical nurse specialists, certified nurse practitioners, certified nurse–midwives, and certified registered nurse anesthetists. Formal peer review processes and structures for APRNs promotes practice autonomously, self-regulation, continuous professional development, risk management, and the full application of APRN advanced knowledge and skills. Promoting clinical effectiveness and evidence-based practice, APRN peer review also supports the efforts to advance APRN independent practice as a norm rather that an exception (ANA, 2008). The APRN peer review is applicable to both hospital-employed and hospital-privileged APRNs.

Establishing an APN shared governance council is one new approach being implemented to address APRN peer review, quality, practice advancement, and professional development issues. Participation and representation of all APRNs practicing within an organization, regardless of employment arrangement, can be included in the APN Council activities. Combining all APRN roles across practice settings provides a substantial peer review group, provides cross specialty sharing of knowledge and skills, and helps advance the practice of nursing overall. Presentations of prepared case studies by the APN who were involved in care are typical at these meetings to enhance learning and obtain peer feedback. The case review model emphasizes individual professional accountability to maintain optimum standards of practice using critical and reflective practice evaluation. Case reviews facilitate professional development to improve the quality of care provided.

Additionally, a smaller subcommittee of APRNs is needed to advance the credentialing and privileging process of all APRNs. A sample administration policy for APN credentialing and privileging is provided in Figure 5-7.

## THE NURSING MANAGEMENT COUNCIL

The NMC is accountable for all resources both human and fiscal. This group also is responsible for reward and recognition, excellence in performance outcomes, the hiring of exemplary employees, and corrective action for consistent poor performance. Each member of the management team is held responsible by the management council to define and implement decisions made by the council.

Manager-to-manager peer review can help ensure the consistency in the application of evidence-based decisions made by the NMC. Ideal areas for peer review for practice advancement include unit-based quality, safety, and financial data, employee satisfaction shared leadership practices, and transformational leadership behaviors. Helpful resources regarding national leadership competencies are available in the ANA's *Nursing Administration: Scope and Standards of Practice* (2009) and *AONE Guiding Principles for the Role of the Nurse Executive in Patient Safety* (American Organization of Nurse Executives, 2007).

Manager-to-manager feedback and problem solving can enhance the quality of practice, as its does with direct care nurses. Several examples of manager peer review in advancing the evidence-based practice are presented here.

### Housewide Peer Review Using Nursing Satisfaction

The NMC routinely reviews the nurse satisfaction data for all the areas of nursing practice. In one such review of the housewide and unit-level data, they recognize that one unit is considerably below the standard of the benchmarked hospitals in the sample for nursing satisfaction. There is also one unit that is considerably above the benchmark. To foster learning and support the manager with the lower score, the NMC recommends that the two units' managers

**Figure 5-7.  Administrative policy for APN credentialing and privileging.**

**Subject:** The credentialing and privileging for advanced practice nurses (APRN)
**Purpose:** To establish criteria and processes for APRN applications to the Discipline of Nursing for credentialing and appointment of privileges in a healthcare system setting.
Procedure for clinical privileges:

1. Credentialing will permit the APRN to perform those patient care functions with respect to core privileges outlined in the list of treatments and other diagnostics tests that are based on what the APRN is qualified, licensed, and credentialed to perform as determined by basic educational standards. The APRN will seek privileges based on state law and on the basis of collaborative practice agreements with physicians as determined by medical staff bylaws and institutional policies.
2. The APRN will practice within the specific professional responsibilities and hospital policies identified with an authorized scope of practice. APRNs may apply for additional privileges based on additional knowledge or experience before or during the recredentialing process, which shall occur every 2 years.
3. Clinical privileges for APRNs shall be based on the applicant's education, training, experience, demonstrated current competence, references, and peer review.
4. Additional requirements for performance are determined by the APN Council. Such criteria shall include, but not be limited to the following: role of advancing the practice within nursing, participation in the APRN peer review program, attendance at all required meetings of the APN group as all annual meetings of the nursing discipline, educational presentations, and student mentorship programs.
5. The APN Council will review all validation documents and request for privileges. These forms are initiated by the APRN and forwarded to the APN Council chair upon completion.
6. The APRN will receive a full set of nursing bylaws upon acceptance into the discipline.
7. The completed and approved file of the APRN will be sent by the chair of the APN Council to the CNO who will forward on to the medical staff chair for the completion of the collaborative practice agreement.
8. The APN Council chair and the CNO will both present the candidates at the board-level approval process meetings.
9. The APRN will receive a letter from the APN Council accepting their application and granting privileges after the board decisional process occur.
10. Orientation to the role and role expectations of the nursing shared governance structure are explained at this point, and APRN is assigned to work committees as appropriate. The APRN is now listed on the nursing Web page as consultant in their area of expertise.

meet to collaborate and share best practices ideas. Mentorship is a well-defined evidence-based intervention. The NMC also requires the mentor manager to assist the other manager to develop a goal and action plan. During this process, the mentor role models how to be transparent with the data in staff and council meetings by engaging the staff in joint problem solving and shared decision making. The actions taken to move forward and improve nurse satisfaction belong to the mentored manager and the unit leadership.

### Unit-Level Peer Review Using Hours per Patient Day

Annually, the NMC determines the nursing budget and hours per patient day (HPPD) for all units based on the national standards and in accordance with professional associations staffing guidelines. The nursing care delivery system and response to regulatory requirements are defined at the unit level. In the NMC routine monitoring of the staff effectiveness, it is determined that one unit is considerably above the national benchmark in HPPD, at a significant cost to the nursing budget. The NMC asks the unit-level manager to the review care delivery system with their unit-based practice council to determine reasons for this budget variance and to create an action plan. In collaboration with the manager, the unit-based practice council determines that a unique patient population exists on their unit, of frail elderly patients age 85 and older. The manager and the unit-based Practice Council determine that there is no national benchmark data on HPPD for this patient population. The manager reports back to the NMC that the unit-based practice council plans to research this area more fully and report back to the NMC. They engage finance, human resources, and productivity specialists in discovering this new knowledge.

### Peer Review in Organizations with Collective Bargaining Agreements

Often the question of whether peer review can be done in organizations where the nurses are represented by a third-party collective bargaining organization comes up for discussion. The following rules of engagement have been found to be successful in organizations:

- The peer review structure should be sanctioned by the collective bargaining agreement between hospital and nurse. It is important to include the union representation in the development and design of the shared governance and peer review structures.
- Peer review within shared governance councils is created to accomplish professional issues only and should not deal with issues concerning grievances, labor disputes, wages, rates of pay, hours, or other terms of (and conditions of) employment.

- The peer review process, once designed, is written into the collective bargaining agreement so that both parties have decisional powers.
- Any shared governance structure including peer review cannot impede the rights of an individual nurse to use the contractual grievance process.
- Peer review, granting of credentials, and other professional issues of advancement are proper areas of authority for councils if authorized in bylaws that have been approved by both parties. The decisions and recommendations of the peer review councils should be relevant, reasonable, and done in good faith with honesty through objective criteria.

First and foremost, there must be a strong nursing shared governance structure, which clearly supports direct care nurses involvement in decision making around the issues of practice and professional image. The governance structure is used as a framework for getting the work done with direct care nurse engagement and involvement at all levels, and is sanctioned in the union contract.

Management must be supportive of and very clear in discerning what decisions are management decisions and what are staff governance decisions. Leadership must coach and educate the direct care nurses and the union representatives in how to manage those issues related to professionalism and practice parameters. This creates a level of autonomy for staff and management. For example, many organizations have adopted the concept of peer interviewing following appropriate education and competency validation for participants. Peer interviewing can be an autonomous practice of the staff. Staff must recognize, however, that only management can offer the candidate employment in positions. Proper education of all parties is critical before implementing any peer review process.

When working with union organizations, a clear differentiation between the performance evaluation done by the manager and the peer review done by the staff is essential. When the union understands that peer review is a way to improve quality and safety, and their members facilitate the process amongst the peer group, there is less resistance to adoption. In this environment, managers and union representation begin to develop a trusting relationship because the union understands that the feedback aspect of peer review is always being done in a nonpunitive, coaching way by the staff and it is not included in the performance evaluation process.

Role advancement in the form of clinical ladders that include a monetary reward is always a bargaining item. Planning must be done for this form of peer review in order to include the union representatives early on in the design and implementation process, as well as for the development of the language for the bargaining agreement.

Another use of the peer review process is to empower nurses to handle issues of practice and professionalism that are focused on quality and safety. The hospital and union must recognize that there are outcomes for improvement that must be met from both a regulatory and a patient satisfaction perspective. Nurses as professionals are bound by a professional code of ethics that also guide their practice. Specifically, the Code of Ethics for Nurses calls for nurses to participate "in establishing, maintaining and improving health care environments and conditions of employment conducive to the provision of quality health care and consistent with the values of the profession through individual and collection action" (ANA, 2001, p. 20). It also states that "the profession of nursing, as represented by associations and their members, is responsible for articulating nursing values, for maintaining the integrity of the profession and its practices, and shaping social policy" (p. 24). It is important for direct care nurses, managers, and the union to understand that nursing as a discipline is held accountable to the entire code of ethics for nursing and to the tenets of professionalism, including peer review. Because peer review is the major element that has been undeveloped, this is the work that needs to be advanced collectively using the principles of partnership, ownership, equity, and accountability. These concepts must be played out in the context of transformational leadership in the healthcare system.

## REFERENCES

Almada, P., Carafoli, K., Flattery, J. B., French, D. A., & McNamara, M. (2004). Improving the retention rate of newly graduated nurses. *Journal for Nurses in Staff Development, 20*(6), 268–273.

American Association of Critical-Care Nurses. (2005). *AACN standards for establishing and sustaining healthy work environments.* Aliso Viejo, CA: Author.

American Nurses' Association. (1988). *Peer review guidelines.* Kansas City, MO: Author.

American Nurses' Association. (2001). *Code of ethics for nurses with interpretive statements.* Silver Spring, MD: Author.

American Nurses' Association. (2008). *Guide to the code of ethic for nurses: Interpretation and application.* Silver Spring, MD: Nursebooks.org.

American Nurses' Association. (2009). *Nursing administration: Scope and standards of practice.* Silver Spring, MD: Author.

American Organization of Nurse Executives. (2007). *The AONE guiding principles of the role of the nurse executive in patient safety.* Chicago, IL: Author.

American Society of PeriAnesthesia Nurses. (2002). *Clinical guidelines for the prevention of unplanned perioperative hypothermia.* Cherry Hill, NJ: Author.

American Society of PeriAnesthesia Nurses. (2007). Position statement 11. Available at: http://www.aspan.org/Portals/6/docs/ClinicalPractice/PositionStatement/11-Visitation_Ph_I.pdf. Accessed January 18, 2010.

Anderson, D., & Webster, C. (2001). A systems approach to the reduction of medication error on the hospital ward. *Journal of Advanced Nursing, 34*(1), 43–41.

Barnum, B. S. (1996). Foreword. In P. Benner, C. A. Tanner, & C. A. Chesla (Eds.), *Expertise in nursing practice: Caring, clinical judgment and ethics.* New York, NY: Springer.

Benner, P. (1984). *From novice to expert.* Menlo Park, CA: Addison-Wesley.

BFHI USA. (2010). *Implementing the UNICEF/WHO baby friendly hospital initiative in the U.S.* Available at http://www.babyfriendlyusa.org/eng/index.html. Accessed January 12, 2010.

Dossey, B. M., Selanders, L. C., Beck, D.-M., & Attewell, A. (2005). *Florence Nightingale today: Healing, leadership, global action.* Silver Spring, MD: nursebooks.org.

Evans, B. (2005). Best practice protocols: VAP prevention. *Nursing Management, 36*(12), 10–16.

Fiddler, M., Marienau, C., & Whitaker, U. (2006). *Assessing learning: Standards, principles & procedures* (2nd ed.). Dubuque, IA: Kendall/Hunt.

Gray, S. (1999). Metro clinical practice development model: Redesign for the region. In B. Haag-Heitman (Ed.), *Clinical practice development using novice to expert theory* (pp. 175–194). Gaithersburg, MD: Aspen.

Haag-Heitman, B. (2008). The development of expert performance in nursing. *Journal for Nurses in Staff Development, 24*(5), 203–211.

Haag-Heitman, B. (Ed). (1999). *Clinical practice development using novice to expert theory.* Gaithersburg, MD: Aspen.

Harrington, L. (2009). Hardwiring nursing quality. *Nurse Leader, 7*(2), 44–46.

Institute for Healthcare Improvement (2007). *Prevent ventilator-associated pneumonia.* Available at http://www.ihi.org/IHI/Programs/Campaign/VAP.htm. Accessed October 7, 2009.

Porter-O'Grady, T. (1985). Credentialing, privileging, and nursing bylaws: Assuring accountability. *Journal of Nursing Administration, 15*(12), 23–27.

Porter-O'Grady, T. (2009). Health care in a quantum age. In T. Porter-O'Grady (Ed.), *Interdisciplinary shared governance: Integrating practice, transforming health care* (2nd ed., pp. 1–38). Sudbury, MA: Jones and Bartlett.

Ringerman, E., Flint, L., & Hughes, D. (2006). An innovative education program: Peer competency validation model. *Journal for Nurses in Staff Development, 22*(3), 114–121.

Santucci, J. (2004). Facilitating the transition into nursing practice: Concepts and strategies for mentoring new graduates. *Journal for Nurses in Staff Development, 20*(6), 274–284.

Schmidt, L., Nelson, D., & Godfrey, L. (2003). A clinical ladder program based on Carper's fundamental patterns of knowing in nursing. *Jurnal of Nursing Administration, 33*(3), 146–152.

Senge, P., Kleiner, A., Roberts, C., Ross, R., & Smith, B. (1994). *The fifth discipline fieldbook.* New York, NY: Doubleday Dell.

Tanner, C. (2006). Thinking like a nurse: a research-based model of clinical judgment in nursing. *Journal of Nursing Education, 45*(6), 204–211.

The Joint Commission (2008). *Accreditation program: Hospital national patient safety goals.* Available at http://www.jointcommission.org/NR/rdonlyres/31666E86-E7F4-423E-9BE8-F05BD1CB0AA8/0/HAP_NPSG.pdf. Accessed October 15, 2009.

Valentine, P. (1995). Management of conflict: Do nurses/women handle it differently? *Journal of Advanced Nursing, 22*(1), 142–149.

Williams, S. C. (1996). *Expert and non-expert nurses' perspectives of life experiences related to becoming and being a nurse* (Unpublished doctoral dissertation). University of South Carolina, Columbia, SC.

# CHAPTER 6

# Shared Leadership Education: Preparing the Staff to Lead in Peer Review

The concept of shared leadership is a new paradigm for healthcare organizations. As organizations change from bureaucratic structures of decision making, to processes that encourage the knowledge worker to be empowered to make decisions at the point of service, a new definition of leadership must emerge. Managers who work in these new healthcare systems must be transformational and learn new ways of sharing responsibilities for the decisions made with both their professional and nonprofessional staff. Shared leadership demands a new set of skills for both management and staff.

## SECURING THE RESOURCES

Shared leadership training requires an ongoing long-term financial investment in developing direct care staff, the management team, APRNs, and educators. Providing education and professional development opportunities in the clinical setting means not only time and attention to the educational processes, but also the need to plan into the budget the monies for release time for staff to learn and practice. This planning should be included in the strategic plan for nursing so that valuable resources of money and education time can be prioritized and used to build the skills necessary for staff management, and other nurse leaders to lead in this new paradigm. The type of leadership needed to facilitate the staff's use of autonomous decision-making skills while leading in changing culture is defined by Yukl (1994) as a leader who is able to influence the follower toward a common purpose or to accomplish a particular task. Literature from several different disciplines was used to design the concepts for shared leadership training presented in this chapter such that they would demonstrate an administrative evidence-based practice.

## SYSTEM'S THEORY APPROACH

Ford (1992) described a systems approach to behavioral change and achievement that balances variables of motivation, acquisition of skill, and a responsive environment. These elements are described in Chapter 2 under the conceptual framework for peer review behavioral change. The shared leadership model of training uses these elements of the framework. The concepts of adult learning theory and leadership goal/feedback theory is described in more detail as they become critical to the personal success of the individual's growth and learning around these processes. As shown in the conceptual framework described in Chapter 2, the process of behavioral change for direct care RNs is complex and multivariate. As the process of behavioral change begins to take shape and direct care staff accept a leadership role in a peer review process, the culture begins to change. The implementation of a variety of peer review strategies will be necessary to produce the desired outcomes of accountability and patient care quality and safety.

## RESEARCH ON LEADERSHIP: WHY CHANGE?

### Moving from Industrial Age Leadership

During the 20th century, management underwent a significant transformation in beliefs and behaviors. As a result of this transformation, many aspects of the business enterprise also began changing. The once accepted definition of effective management written about by Frederick Taylor in the 1920s, described the manager's success in terms of the hierarchic control over decision making that leads to profitable outcomes. The boss at the top made all the decisions, and the workers simply carried them out. This model appeared to have success during the industrial age as the workforce, many who were transplanted agricultural workers who had moved into cities during the industrial revolution. These workers were often craftsmen, now doing production work. Another set of workers during this time represented displaced immigrants who had traveled to America. Both of these groups of workers were not educated in management, many lacked the skills of reading and writing, and were therefore ill prepared to lead change. Most of what was decided by business management was top-down and written in memos, policies, and procedure manuals, those workers who wanted to advance in the workforce needed communications skills as well.

## MOVING INTO THE KNOWLEDGE AGE

As the workers developed, and the social and political environments changed, so did the workforce. The workforce, now educated in colleges and universities, has become the most knowledgeable in the history of our world. We have moved succinctly into the information age because the workforce developed the skill set necessary to move us there. Managers now yield to a different model of decision making called participatory management. Participatory management is more flexible and is more open to employee initiatives. Although this form of management may be moving us closer to the model needed for the future, much of the workforce still finds it too controlling. In participatory management, managers are still directing the work of the employee. As concepts of developing customer loyalty through satisfaction engage the new business enterprise and profits are made through innovation and creativity from the workforce, a new model of management must emerge. Employee empowerment and engagement are the essential new measures leading to organizational success (Bell & Zemke, 1992; Manz & Sims, 1987; Saunders, 1995).

Shared leadership is the term used to describe the new partnership behaviors needed for effective management working with knowledge workers. The leader acts not from his or her power role of directing and controlling, but through motivating the workforce around a goal or task that must be met. Shared leadership occurs within the context of a social system (Yukl, 1994). The literature examines this style of leadership as a shared phenomenon between the manager and the follower.

## SYNOPSIS OF LEADERSHIP THEORIES

Several researchers have attempted to define the term of leadership. Hemphill and Coons (1957) wrote that leadership is the behavior of an individual when he is directing the activity of a group toward a shared goal. Tannenbaum, Weschler, and Massarik (1961) defined leadership as interpersonal influence, exercised in a situation, and directed through a communication process toward the attainment of a specific set of goals. Yukl (1994) suggested that these differences in definition and means of measurement lead to a variety of phenomena for investigation and to a myriad of recommendations for the development of the management practitioner. An individual's practice in management was led by the genre of leadership theories to which the practitioner subscribed. These are described in broad categories as trait theory, the behavioral approach, the power and influence paradigm, and transactional to transformational theory.

### Trait Theory

Researchers in the 1930s and 1940s, conducted many studies to assess the traits that differentiated great leaders from nonleaders. Through reviewing all of these studies, Stogdill (1948) concluded that one does not become a leader by virtue of possessing some common set of traits, but rather, the leader emerges as he or she bears some relevant relationship to the characteristics, activities, and goals of the follower. After again reviewing some 163 trait studies done between 1940 and 1970, Stogdill recognized that the traits of leadership were absolutely necessary for effective leadership. The traits included adaptability to situations, being alert to the social environment, and being ambitious and results oriented. He also describes the leader as being assertive, cooperative, decisive, dependable, and self-confident. The skills a successful leader needed to develop included being creative, socially skilled, and able to tolerate stress while assuming responsibility.

## The Behavioral Approach

The behavioral approach emerged as researchers became discouraged with trait theory and began to pay attention to what managers actually do on the job. Mintzberg (1979) developed the first taxonomy of 10 managerial roles for coding the content of all activities of the leaders' position, duties, and responsibilities. Some of these roles included figurehead, leader, and liaison. Stewart (1998) found that behavior could be classified according to three components. The first related to relationships and how managers handle demands through building relationships. The second had to do with the type of work pattern, that is, whether the work was self-generated or emerged from the work of others. The third relates to the type of work exposure or amount of responsibility one needed to make decisions. The work of the behavioral approach researchers summarizes the skills need for managers. These skills include the ability to define roles and establish superior/subordinate relationships, the ability to take risks and problem solve by getting and giving information according to work load, and the ability to influence others thorough a common purpose of health, life, or organizational success.

## Power and Influence Approach

Influence, some researchers have asserted, is the essence of power. Power is the capacity to exert influence through leadership. The manner in which power is enacted also influences behavior. Dansereau and Yammarino (1998) suggested that effective leaders, those whose results end in group success, not only have a strong influence over followers but are actually receptive to the followers influence on them as well. Although these authors did not use the term "shared leadership," they empirically began to describe its effects.

Yukl and Tracey (1992) conducted two studies with different research methods and proposed that the effectiveness of an influence tactic depended on five aspects of the situation. These were: (1) the amount of intrinsic resistance by the target because of nature of the request, (2) the potential of the tactic to influence the target attitudes about the desirability of the requested action, (3) the agent's possession of an appropriate power base for use of the tactics in that context, (4) the agent skill in using the tactic, and (5) the prevailing social norms and role expectations about the use of the tactic. The end result was that the participant's commitment to accomplish the task and the autonomy the follower possessed over the course of the task emerged as two critical variables.

### Transactional to Transformational Theory

In Burns and Stalkner's (1961) transformational leadership paradigm, the leader raised the follower's awareness to the importance and value of goals, and helped determine how to reach them. They asserted that through this process, the leader influenced the follower to transcend his or her own self-interest for the sake of the team or organization. The transformational leader, unlike the transactional leader, identifies and articulates a shared vision, provides the appropriate structural model, fosters the acceptance of group goals, and has high performance expectations. During this process of attaining goals, the leader provides individualized support and consideration while offering intellectual stimulation and allowing self-actualization to occur. Transformational leadership underscores the importance of the follower's role and understands the critical nature of the interaction between the leader and the follower. Most research has favored this type of leadership, and in fact, the ANCC Magnet Recognition Program (American Nurses Credentialing Center, 2008) promotes this form of leadership as the first component of the newly revised Magnet model.

## SHARED LEADERSHIP AND EMPOWERMENT: THE NEW MODEL OF LEADERSHIP

Dansereau and Yammarino (1998) advise that the role of leader does not rest with those in positions of power and legitimate influence, but is a role inherent in each of us. If multidirectional and reciprocal influence is necessary to affect outcomes in organizations, then leadership actions are required from all members of the organization. This proposition would assert that each individual, if given the appropriate prescription of skills development, can perform as an effective leader. This would is the foundation for structure empowerment. According to Yukl (1994), shared responsibility for leadership functions and empowerment is more effective when everyone believes that the expectation for delivery of all successful outcomes does not rest solely with the manager. The extent to which the leadership can be shared effectively is predicated on the organizational conditions that facilitate the process, and the importance the organization places on the individual's performance in this arena.

Bass (1990), in his landmark paper on transformational leadership, suggested that there is a universality to this leadership style and he closely links it by description with the concept of shared leadership. This new leadership model does not replace the previously described theories on leadership but actually extends the model to include a new role called the transformational leader. In this new role, the leader shares in leading by adopting a philosophy of transparency and a sharing of information. Bass asserts that this model of transactional to transformational leadership can be extended to expand the follower's behaviors through building relationships while focusing on changes in motivation, sense of understanding, maturity, and self-worth. Outcomes of transformational leadership are engaged in as the follower shares in the leader's activities. The educational paradigm for leadership is clear. It requires the development of skills that can negotiate mutually agreed upon team outcomes, solve problems in complex environments, and motivate human behavior.

### Leadership in Heath Care and Nursing

This approach to shared leadership demands a responsive healthcare environment of leaders. Leadership in health care is needed to respond to the complex integrated systems that are emerging out of the growth and restructuring of the typical community hospital or the tertiary academic healthcare environment. All professionals, including nurses, must embrace the concept and be educated on the skill set of transformational leadership to improve the outcomes for those served.

Nursing leadership literature has evolved over the past 100 years as well. Within nursing, however, little has been written about effective teaching strategies to develop the empowered workforce. In a 1994 editorial, Mattera made a distinction between being a nurse manager or administrator and being a leader. She noted that staff nurses required information about leadership as it occurred at the bedside. Nurses, she noted, needed help in communicating, seeing, and understanding the context of nursing care from a broader perspective if they were to understand their patients' issues. Sams (1996) wrote a commentary after experiencing leadership training and noted two very important lessons. She indicated that in her view, leadership skills were essential for team building, creative thinking, and reflective practice. These skills helped her to see what is realistic without losing the overall vision, allowed her to acknowledge resource limitation without losing the ability to negotiate for more, and made her aware of the social and political changes that affect nursing practice in an organized setting. This set of skills helped her to reframe obstacles as possibilities.

A few researchers have conducted studies that evaluate leadership continuing education programs. Waddell (1992) published a meta-analysis of continuing education on nursing practice, although not specific to leadership development. It demonstrated that continuing education has a positive impact on nursing practice. Two other studies from the literature could be seen as instructive in designing a model of leadership education for staff. Brock (1978) described the results of teaching a 1-month management course to 80 senior BSN students. Findings revealed that leadership values held by nursing students did not affect their leadership behaviors. However, students who took a leadership course demonstrated significantly more leadership behaviors after having taken the course. Krejci and Malin (1997) demonstrated that self-perceived leadership understanding and ability increased after leadership training.

Although training certainly helps to develop leadership skills, training alone will not change staff nurses' behaviors completely. Dwyer, Schwartz, and Fox (1992) assessed that any program on leadership should emphasize the nurse's need for high levels of autonomy and the need for feedback that consists of recognition and support for individual preferences and strengths. Dwyer *et al.* concluded that teaching needed to include workshops designed to increase self-awareness and to provide feedback on performance. They indicated that a demonstrated rate of increased autonomy would have a positive impact on patient care. A major element of the shared leadership training program described in the following section was the clear assumption that if you taught staff nurses leadership skills, returned them to an environment responsive to practicing these skills, and provided a self-awareness feedback tool for performance, that staff nurses would increase their level of professional autonomy.

## Research on Shared Leadership Training

Shared leadership training builds a skill set for direct care nurses that when used in practice can lead to increased leadership skills and professional practice autonomy. Research has demonstrated that when staff nurses are educated about the concepts of negotiation, systems thinking, empowerment, facilitation, and accountability, staff demonstrated higher levels of professional autonomy (George, 1999). Maas and Jacox's research (1977) confirmed that a clear relationship exists between the quality of the service provided by nurses and the extent to which they perceive themselves as able to function autonomously in decision making concerning their practice. Aiken, Smith, and Lake (1994) and Aiken, Sochalski, and Lake (1997) reaffirmed this assertion when they demonstrated that nurses affect patient outcomes by their direct action (independent practice) and their influence over others (peer review). They also suggested that patients were positively affected when the model of leadership resulted in greater nurse autonomy and control of practice, and improvement at the point of care.

### *Components of the Shared Leadership Training Program*

As CNO, George (1999) facilitated a shared leadership training program in her organization. To meet the stated objectives of this learning design, leadership abilities were culled from a variety of evidence-based administrative and learning practices research (Kouzes & Posner, 1987; Porter-O'Grady & Wilson, 1998;

Senge, Kleiner, Roberts, Ross, & Smith, 1994; Yukl, 1994). These included the ability to negotiate to a win-win solution through team learning, facilitating change in self and others through good communication skills (listening, giving and receiving feedback); through thinking and problem solving in a systems framework; and by empowering others to act responsibility through a shared vision and decision making process. These elements comprise the primary components of the shared leadership training program and are described further in this chapter.

### Creating the Shared Vision for Leadership Training

Evaluation of the evidence-based leadership training program reported by George (1999) guides this section. Before embarking on the implementation of a shared leadership training program that will involve the direct care RNs, it is important to engage with shared governance leaders. The chief nursing officer (CNO) should initiate a conversation with staff leaders in the shared governance structure through a strategic planning session. Reviewing the evidence-based practice of the training program will help focus the planning. Elements of control over the education process should be developed and should conceptually appear in the nursing strategic plan. The operational elements and financing of the process should appear in the operational plans for the organization and therefore should also appear in the managers, and directors, personal goals. This will give the discipline of nursing ownership over all goals to accomplish over a set time frame. It also defines which shared governance council (e.g., the Professional Development and Education Council) should take control of the process and manage all the design decisions. The nursing strategic plan should set forth a framework for individual and unit goal setting by unit-based councils at the local level.

Once the organization-wide councils have made their decisions, unit-level councils must meet to define their local level goals in alignment with the criteria set forth by the organization-wide councils. Each unit council can define the operational plan needed to meet these goals at the local level. The time frame for completion of the goals at the unit level needs to coincide with the organization-wide timeline.

It is important that those who will be doing the coaching, mentoring, and development of goals with the staff all have shared leadership skills and have attended this course of study. Management and clinical staff leaders, including the shared governance members and advanced practice nurses (APNs), should go through the program first. All leaders would then role model the shared leadership behaviors learned in their respective units. The shared accountability for applying the new concepts is one of the key strategies to organization-wide success.

## Goal Development and Feedback Theory

The identification of learning goals before training is the second key strategy to the individual learner's success. The beneficial effect of goal setting on task performance is one of the most robust and replicable findings in the psychological literature (Yukl & Latham, 1978). Goal and feedback theory would suggest that the strongest motivation patterns are those anchored in the personal and professional goals of the individual. Goals must constantly meet the optimal challenge of the individual. In the context of the workplace, the goal setting process should connect the goals of the person to the goals of the organization. This congruence leads to recognition of accomplishments by the person/employee through intrinsic rewards, as well as those extrinsic rewards fostered by the organization.

The third strategy to the individual's learning success is the use of open and honest feedback about goals attainment and expectations for performance. Yukl and Latham (1978) showed that knowledge of the results alone was not sufficient to improve performance and that knowledge of performance and goal setting for results did increase performance. The level at which the goals were set was influenced by feedback about prior performance. Quiñones (1995) suggested that the framing of training assignments and feedback from previous training assignments formed a different attitudinal and motivational perspective going into the next training program. He also found that when the need for training was framed for the trainee before going into training, it affected motivation and performance. Self-efficacy perceptions of the trainee resulted in higher motivation to actually learn.

Yukl and Latham (1978) asserted that when employees have substantial influence in setting goals, employee traits and values affect the difficulty of the perceived goal. The need for achievement was one trait likely to affect one's perception of the goal's difficulty. A high need achiever tended to set a moderately difficult goal and tended to revise the goal upward after it has been attained. This would indicate an increase in performance. Participation in goal setting resulted in goal acceptance and commitment when there was a strong need for achievement and autonomy, and when an individual possessed high self-esteem and internal locus of control. These researchers found that employees with a strong need for independence have great goal acceptance when their participation in the goal setting process was increased. Goals affect performance by directing attention, mobilizing personal effort, and increasing persistence as a motivating strategy develops.

In the context of the workplace, staff who are selected for this training process should meet with the manager and unit-based APN to establish a set of personal- and unit-specific goals that would be applied at the conclusion of the shared leadership training series. In addition, it is important that staff be told about expectations for the feedback process and should recognize the need for reflection on this feedback during the educational series. For example, a staff nurse might develop with his or her manager that at the conclusion of the shared leadership training series, they will run for a unit- or organization-wide council seat in shared governance to apply their new leadership skills. Another area for goal development is leading a TIPS process on their unit to improve patient safety outcomes.

### Feedback from Peers and Leaders

The leadership practices inventory (LPI) is a tool nationally and internationally recognized to assess observed leadership behaviors (Kouzes & Posner, 1987). It is a valid and reliable tool that, when used with staff or management, can provide the data necessary for reflection and growth. It also provides a set of data that will help learners to determine what areas of continued leadership education they should pursue. The LPI tool should be given to all participants in the program before classes start and then again at the conclusion of the program. These results are kept confidential between the participants and their coach, who helps the participant to review and interpret the data, as well as set future goals.

### Who Are the Teachers?

The teachers in the shared leadership program need to be from all roles of nursing in the organization, such as direct care nurses, APRNs, educators, and managers. It is important in adult learning theory that the trainers be action oriented and adept at telling their own personal stories of leadership development. It is recommended that all levels of nursing be involved in the teaching, as each role brings a unique experience to the education table. As staff nurses become increasingly adept at these leadership behaviors, they, in turn, become influential teachers for others.

It is well documented in the communication literature that stories help create shared meaning and inclusion. Stories can be powerful teaching methods and must come from the heart of the teacher. Stories have given us a mechanism to talk to one another across a rich and diverse medium we call nursing. Nurses are natural storytellers, and are in a constant habit of testing whether the stories they hear ring true with the stories they know to be true as experienced in their own lives. In this teaching framework, leaders from all levels explore with staff from their own experiences in leading and demonstrating clinical stories of autonomy at the bedside. Managers can influence attendees to grow as leaders by using stories from their own practice and by describing their own journeys to becoming leaders. APRNs and educators tell a different story of becoming a leader. The CNO/directors teach from a perspective of defined role authority of leader and learn from these stories of empowerment and, in turn, experience how those elements of direct care nurses stories influence their own leadership style.

**The Responsive Environment**

It is imperative that the environment into which the learner returns supports the concepts of the learning received (Tracey, Tannenbaum, & Kavanagh, 1995; Troyan, 1996). Following shared leadership training, direct care nurses must see a level of demonstrated commitment by those in formal leadership roles. It is imperative for leaders to create an environment that is supportive of the shared leadership process, and values the demonstration of the newly acquired leadership skills of negotiating, facilitating, empowering, and giving feedback (peer review). Empirical outcomes from shared leadership training are reported in a study conducted by George, Burke, and Rogers (1999). Participants reported both personal self-growth, and perceptions of meeting their patients' needs more often after training. These nurses also indicated feedback from their patients expressing trust and satisfaction with their care. Additionally, they reported that they were able to teach the patient and family how to negotiate the healthcare system more effectively. And finally, they felt teamwork was improved, and they were increasingly more attentive to RN/MD relations and peer satisfaction.

To ensure consistency in the leadership framework application, the manager/APRN/educator must attend the same series of shared leadership educational programs, feedback sessions, and goal setting with his or her superiors, as their staff did. Engaging the entire discipline of nursing in shared leadership training helps ensure alignment and uniformity in expectations across all practice areas.

**Presenting the Program**

The shared leadership training program should be presented over a period of 3 to 6 months to give participants opportunities to apply the new learning in their normal practice. To create, build, and sustain momentum, it is recommended that the educational sessions are scheduled 1 to 2 months apart, in 4 to 8 hour sessions. When the participant returns to the classroom, they explore their experiences applying the shared leadership concepts with other participants. This planned educational intervention affords a good opportunity for the organization to conduct their own research to demonstrate behavioral changes in leadership, autonomy, and patient outcomes. Because research has demonstrated that it takes 12 to 18 months to see human behavioral change (George, 1999), this would be a longitudinal study and should be identified as a research priority in the nursing strategic plan.

**Professionalism of Peer Review**

Professionalism for all disciplines requires a unique body of knowledge, the establishment of a collective for decision making, a peer review process, and the professional's need to serve the client in an autonomous, but still accountable, means. A formal structure of shared leadership training is one mechanism that can enhance development of the behaviors necessary to carry out the professional work of the nursing discipline. Any discipline that chooses to take a leadership role within an organizational context can also benefit from similar shared leadership training.

By being clear around the definition of the role of the nurse and the expected measurable outcomes of accountability of the discipline, nursing can take its leadership seat at the decisional table with all the other clinical disciplines. Together, the members of the interdisciplinary team, all schooled in the roles and accountabilities of being a leader at the point of care, will develop formal and informal methods of communication based on standards of care for each discipline. In combining standards, a structure of decision making for patient care will emerge. Each member of the team will be able to communicate, negotiate for resources, and define the clinical outcomes of his or her unique discipline. These leaders will decide and implement the interdisciplinary governance structure for patient care. They will establish of a set of interdisciplinary standards of care that are measured through each discipline's peer review process. The transformational leaders of tomorrow will set the stage for improvement in care processes of health systems. In the development of healing, wellness-oriented systems of care for the patients and families will be the true measure of our cultural transformation.

### *Program Outcomes for Shared Leadership Development*

Participants in the shared leadership development program will be able to:

- Define accountability and demonstrate accountability-based behaviors in their role, which includes timely confrontation of nonaccountable-type behaviors
- Reframe conflict to one of opportunity in daily practice
- Use the principles of negotiation to create win-win solutions
- Demonstrate skillful communication
- Demonstrate personal mastery skills in giving and receiving feedback
- Assume ownership for the peer review process
- Display sensitivity to self and others, thereby promoting a respectful group process to reach decisions through consensus
- Help create, communicate, and integrate a nursing vision on their unit
- Be able to develop personal and unit goals
- Analyze their own environment, identify opportunities, and collaborate on an action plan to break down barriers and promote a "can do" attitude
- Demonstrate inquiry and respect for the mind map of others and incorporate multiple perspectives toward outcome achievement
- Develop a plan and action strategies to move along a determined professional career path
- Solicit and integrate feedback about personal behaviors into a professional development plan

## Using Shared Leadership to Advance Peer Review

Active participation in and completion of the shared leadership education series by a significant proportion of the staff creates the momentum for developing skilled leadership at the point of service. The shared leadership skills are essential to the actualization of the components of the peer review processes, particularly in the area of skilled communication and the ability to give and receive feedback.

The new age of consumer expectations of high quality and patient safety demands that nursing as a disciplines completes this next chapter and begins to implement a comprehensive model of nursing peer review. As the discipline continues to evolve, the integrated peer review process will encompass a focus on quality and safety, role actualization, and practice advancement. As a result, nurses will utilize their new skill set and showcase the outcomes of their important work through professional autonomy and accountability.

## Structural Empowerment

Research on Magnet hospitals indicates that hospitals who support structural empowerment and transformational leadership processes promote better patient outcomes. Those outcomes include lower mortality rates, greater patient satisfaction, lower levels of burnout, and an increase in overall nurse satisfaction (Laschinger, Wong, McMahon, & Kaufmann, 1999; Laschinger, Almost, & Tuer-Hodes, 2003). These findings support the research on empowering work environments. Social structures like shared governance provide employees with access to information to support and resources to facilitate shared decision making. Opportunities to learn and grow through access to information and new technology are empowering and allow employees to accomplish their work in meaningful ways.

## The Transformational Leader

Successful CNOs recognize that cost-effective, high-quality service and care can only be delivered by a team of highly influential healthcare experts that have a vision and a passion for excellence. Clearly, nursing administrators should ensure that the attributes of professionalism, including peer review, are implemented. The role of the transformational CNO of the future is to facilitate the creation of promising new structures of empowerment that can and will develop this essential piece of the quality equation—new models of peer review. This also necessitates a demand for transformational leadership at the bedside. As an outcome of using peer review, practitioners can deliver excellence in quality outcomes 100% of the time.

With 2.7 million professional nurses in the United States, of whom two thirds work at hospitals, it would appear that the place to begin the change in peer review is in the hands of these nurse leaders in hospital settings. The CNO and the staff leadership, in a partnership model of shared governance, play pivotal roles as the nursing administrator and the professional nurse work together to promote all the aspects of peer review from peer interviewing to clinical advancement. The administrative role is grounded in the principles of evidence-based management and practice. The clinical nursing role is fostered by the essential features of professional nursing showcased in the ethical practice of nursing as a discipline.

The CNO's leadership team and staff leaders must recognize that in their positions, they hold a dual responsibility, one is to the organization as a whole, and the other is to the ethics of the profession. This group of leaders plays a vital role in educating the organization to the needs of the profession to accomplish the goals of the organization and their discipline. It is this shared vision that drives the establishment of a shared leadership framework for peer review.

### Professionalism and Peer Review

The concept of peer review remains a crucial and vital undeveloped portion of nursing discipline's professional development. Nursing as a discipline has well defined and implemented the other tenets of professionalism as seen here. Practitioners are using nursing theorists' contributions to the discipline's body of knowledge to design models of care and new care delivery systems consistent with these conceptual frameworks. Evidence-based practice is becoming a common language within the realm of clinical practice discussions, supporting nursing practice standards and driving improvements in nursing care. Shared governance has been in the literature since the 1980s and is experiencing renewed interest in the context of self-regulation. Its principles of equity, ownership, partnership, and accountability have taken on new meaning in the content of practice autonomy and governance. The novice-to-expert continuum is routinely used as a framework for understanding the nursing professional development. An emphasis on individual advancement is taking on new directions in the context of lifelong learning, advancing degrees and certification rates, and moving from licensure and competency testing to credentialing and privileging for nurses at all levels. Technology is leading us into new areas of education with the emergence of online learning, clinical simulation labs, and global connections. Dr. Tim Porter-O'Grady, a contemporary of nursing shared governance development, asked a very important question in 1999 that is still pertinent today. The question for every nurse is: "Who am I and what do I have to contribute to the obligations of my profession and the needs of those we serve?" (Porter-O'Grady, 1999)

### Quality and Patient Safety Outcomes

Patient safety and quality will continue to be a major concern of our society as well as all health-related regulatory bodies. The recent report by the

Institute of Medicine (IOM, 2004) identified nursing as the essential element to the patient safety equation. The IOM report noted that the quality of patient care is directly correlated to the degree to which hospital nurses are active and empowered participants in making decisions about patients' individual plans of care. The vital role of nursing in the delivery of high-quality clinical care and patient's satisfaction with care in the United States has been confirmed by Jha, Orav, Zheng, and Epstein (2008).

An emphasis on the patient's experience and satisfaction with care within the provision of patient-centered care is a key element of high-quality health care (IOM, 2004). Peer review is a critical component to addressing variations and inadequacies in the quality of health care and the healthcare experience across regions and settings. In response to the differences in care and outcomes among hospitals, federal policy makers and private organizations have launched an important program to collect and publicly report data on the quality of the health care Americans receive (Jha *et al.*, 2008). Nursing needs to be proactive in its response to these issues as more and more data on quality and safety continue to be publicly reported. The Hospital Quality Alliance (HQA) program, overseen by private and public entities, including the Centers for Medicare and Medicaid Services (CMS) and The Joint Commission, is leading this effort in the hospital sector, producing quarterly reports on the provision of effective services for common conditions (Jha *et al.*, 2008).

Until recently, there has been little information on the quality of hospital care from patients' perspectives. Data from a Hospital Consumer Assessment of Healthcare Providers and Systems (HCAHPS) survey provides insight into patients' experiences in US hospitals. Summarized in Table 6-1 is the percentage of patients who reported satisfaction with their care on specific HCAHPS components. (Jha *et al.*, 2008, p. 1926).

The domains of patients' experiences in this study, including adequate discharge instructions, nursing services, communication with nurses, and pain control are highly correlated overall. Also significant in the HCAHPS data was the ratio of nurses to patient-days across all characteristics of practice types, location, and patient payor mix. The higher the ratio of nurses to patient-days the more satisfied the patients were, as seen in Table 6-2. The lowest differences were in the areas of physician communication and quietness of the rooms. The authors of this study concluded that,

It is perhaps surprising to note that there was suboptimal performance in areas that have been the target of quality-improvement initiatives for some time. Nearly a third of the patients did not give high ratings in the domain of pain control, despite the focus on this area by the Joint Commission. In addition, despite long-standing interest by the CMS and others in reducing the rate of readmission, many patients did not rate their discharge instructions highly. It is less surprising

**Table 6-1.    Important Elements of Patient Satisfaction**

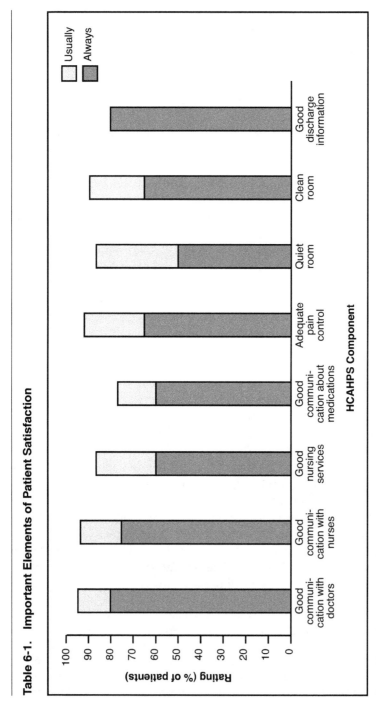

Source: From "Patients' Perception of Hospital Care in the United States," A. K. Jha, E. J. Orav, J. Zheng, and A. M. Epstein, 2008, *The New England Journal of Medicine, 359*, 18, p. 1926. Copyright 2007 by Massachusetts Medical Society. Reprinted with permission.

## Table 6-2.    Effect of Higher Ratio of Nurses on Patient Satisfaction

**Table 2. Percentage of Patients Who Gave a High Global Rating to a Hospital, According to Hospital Characteristics.**

| Characteristic | High Global Rating* | | P Value† |
|---|---|---|---|
| | Unadjusted | Adjusted | |
| | *% of patients* | | |
| **Primary characteristics of interest** | | | |
| Ratio of nurses to patient-days | | | <0.001 |
|     Lowest quartile | 60.1 | 60.5 | |
|     Second quartile | 60.7 | 61.6 | |
|     Third quartile | 64.1 | 64.3 | |
|     Highest quartile | 66.7 | 65.9 | |
| Profit status | | | <0.001 |
|     For-profit | 57.9 | 59.1 | |
|     Not-for-profit, private | 63.6 | 64.8 | |
|     Not-for-profit, public | 65.2 | 65.4 | |
| Academic status‡ | | | 0.51 |
|     Teaching | 63.5 | 63.3 | |
|     Nonteaching | 62.9 | 62.8 | |
| **Other characteristics associated with HCAHPS rating** | | | |
| Location | | | 0.03 |
|     Urban | 62.4 | 62.4 | |
|     Nonurban | 66.7 | 63.7 | |
| Size | | | <0.001 |
|     6–99 beds | 66.4 | 64.8 | |
|     100–399 beds | 61.1 | 62.0 | |
|     ≥400 beds | 63.0 | 62.4 | |
| Census region | | | <0.001 |
|     Northeast | 61.4 | 61.8 | |
|     Midwest | 64.9 | 63.8 | |
|     South | 63.2 | 65.0 | |
|     West | 61.0 | 61.7 | |
| Medical intensive care unit | | | 0.001 |
|     Yes | 62.7 | 62.3 | |
|     No | 63.7 | 63.9 | |
| Medicaid patients | | | <0.001 |
|     Lowest quartile | 65.7 | 65.3 | |
|     Second quartile | 63.5 | 63.1 | |
|     Third quartile | 61.0 | 62.0 | |
|     Highest quartile | 61.5 | 61.9 | |

* A high global rating was defined as a rating of 9 or 10 (on a scale of 0 to 10, with higher scores reflecting better performance) on the Hospital Consumer Assessment of Healthcare Providers and Systems (HCAHPS) survey. In the adjusted analysis, performance on the HCAHPS survey was adjusted for all the other characteristics shown.
† P values are for the results of adjusted analyses.
‡ Academic status was defined according to whether the hospital was a member of the Council of Teaching Hospitals and Health Systems.

to see that communication about medications was often not rated highly, given reports of difficulties with adverse events related to medications. Poor communication at discharge is likely to exacerbate these problems . . . the data presented here provide a comprehensive portrait of patients' experiences in U.S. hospitals. It is clear that the performance of hospitals is variable and that there are plentiful opportunities for improvement. (Jha *et al.*, 2008, pp. 1929–1930)

### Peer Review: The Missing Element

Nursing is recognized as having a central role in healthcare reform and resolving some of the longstanding healthcare issues in this country (Robert Wood Johnson Foundation, 2009). Nursing peer review is the missing element needed to decrease the variability in safety and quality outcomes that plague the US healthcare system. This crisis provides the impetus for nursing to develop dynamic and robust models of peer review to help ensure quality and safety outcomes are achieved. Now, more than ever, nursing must advocate for new and innovative ways to conquer issues related to quality and safety. We need to move beyond ineffective methods such as the historic use of audits for quality monitoring, as these have not provided the level of timely feedback necessary to improve the care outcomes in an ongoing and daily basis. Dynamic forms of peer review is the mechanism for each nurse to take true ownership of his or her practice day by day, shift by shift, and patient by patient. Nurse-to-nurse relationships are enhanced through peer review feedback and provide opportunities for growth along the beginner-to-expert continuum. Patient and nurse relationships will also develop as nurses use partnering techniques to engage patients and families in the care planning process, thereby providing safe and healthy environments. The peer review principles and best practices presented in this book also provide exciting glimpses of how peer review can also enhance organizational partnerships, coalition building, as well as overall communication.

### NEW WORK: INTERDISCIPLINARY PATIENT CARE

Bold action is needed from all disciplines to ensure that health care is safe, high quality, and cost effective. As an essential member of the interdisciplinary team, nursing must actively participate and play a central and active role in decision making, along with other members of the interdisciplinary team. Each nursing participant must be clear and articulate about the unique role that nursing contributes to the patient outcomes and how nursing ensures the quality of contributions through the peer review process. Advancing quality and safety outcomes in an organization demands that members of the interdisciplinary team develop formal and informal methods of communication and decision making. These methods include the creation of interdisciplinary processes for development and evaluation of patient care protocols, identification of shared quality and safety initiatives, patient care conferences and rounding, critical incident reviews, and outcome facilitation teams. In this process, a structure of shared decision making for patient care will emerge.

These are exciting and challenging times for nursing. Moving beyond the current healthcare crisis demands that nursing leaders, both from management and clinical roles, step forward with a high degree of confidence, be courageous, and be willing to take risks in creating a new tomorrow. Creating dynamic peer review processes for nurses at all levels of the organization is an important part of the new leadership order. As with all new processes, the advent of new, system-wide peer review best practices that measures the impact is critical and necessitates research and communication of findings.

Peer review remains the new work of nursing and the work that will frame nursing's future. Assuring quality and safety outcomes using authentic peer review will help maintain our covenant to the public as nursing continues to be rated as the most well-respected, honest, and ethical profession in the eyes of the public (Saad, 2008). The mandate for the future is clear: Nursing must build on that trust by improving quality and patient safety through excellence in nursing practice and peer review.

## REFERENCES

Aiken, L. H., Smith, H. L., & Lake, E. T. (1994). Lower Medicare mortality among a set of hospitals known for good nursing care. *Medical Care, 32*(8), 771–787.

Aiken, L. H., Sochalski, J., & Lake, E. T. (1997). Studying outcomes of organizational change in health services. *Medical Care, 35*(11), NS6–NS18.

American Nurses Association. (2001). *Code of ethics for nurses with interpretive statements.* Silver Spring, MD: Author.

American Nurses Credentialing Center. (2008). *Application manual Magnet recognition program.* Silver Spring, MD: Author.

American Nurses Association. (2009). *Nursing administration: Scope and standards of practice.* Silver Spring, MD: Author.

Bass, B. M. (1990). *Bass and Stogdill's handbook of leadership* (3rd ed.) New York, NY: Free Press.

Bell, C., & Zemke, R. (1998). *Managing knock your socks off service.* New York, NY: Amacom.

Brock, A. M. (1978). Impact of management-oriented course: On knowledge and leadership skills exhibited by Baccalaureate nursing students. *Nursing Research, 27*(4), 271–221.

Burns, T., & Stalkner, G. M. (1961). *The management of innovation.* London, England: Tavistock.

Dansereau, F., & Yammarino, F. J. (Eds.). (1998). Leadership: The multiple-level approaches (Vol. 24). Greenwich, CT: JAI Press.

Dwyer, D., Schwartz, R., & Fox, M. (1992). Decision-making autonomy in nursing. *Journal of Nursing Administration, 22*(2), 17–23.

Ford, M. (1992). *Motivating humans: Goals, emotions, and personal agency beliefs.* Thousand Oaks, CA: Sage Publications.

George, V. (1999). *An organizational case study in shared leadership* (Unpublished doctoral dissertation). Marquette University College of Nursing, Milwaukee, WI.

George, V., Burke. L., & Rogers, B. (1999). *Process and outcomes associated with staff nurse leadership behavior development and use following participation in a shared leadership training program* (Unpublished study). AONE Grant funded by St. Luke's Hospital Medical Center, Milwaukee, WI.

Haag-Heitman, B. (Ed.). (1999). *Clinical practice development using novice to expert theory.* Gaithersburg, MD: Aspen Publishers.

Hemphill, J. K., & Coons, A. E. (1957). Development of the leader behavior description questionnaire. In R. M. Stogdill & A. E. Coons (Eds.), *Leader behavior: Its description and measurement* (pp. 6–38). Columbus, OH: Bureau of Business Research, Ohio State University.

Institute of Medicine (2004). *Keeping patients safe: Transforming the work environment of nurses.* Washington, DC: The National Academics Press

Jha, A. K, Orav, E. J., Zheng, J., & Epstein, A. M. (2008). Patients' perceptions of hospital care in the United States. *The New England Journal of Medicine, 359*(18), 1921–1931.

Kouzes, J. M., & Posner, B. Z. (1987). *The leadership challenge: How to get extraordinary things done in organizations.* San Francisco, CA: Jossey-Bass.

Krejci, J., & Malin, S. (1997). Impact of leadership development on competencies. *Nursing Economics, 15*(5), 235–241.

Laschinger, H., Almost, J., & Tuer-Hodes, D. (2003). Workplace empowerment and magnet hospital characteristics: Making the link. *The Journal of Nursing Administration, 33*(7–8), 410–422.

Laschinger, H., Wong, C., McMahon, L. & Kaufmann, C. (1999). Leader behavior impact on staff nurse empowerment, job tension, and work effectiveness. *The Journal of Nursing Administration, 29*(5), 28–39.

Maas, M., & Jacox, A. (1977). *Guideline for nurse autonomy/patient welfare.* New York, NY: Appleton-Century-Crofts.

Manz, C. & Sims, H. (1987). Leading workers to lead themselves: The external leadership of self-managing work teams. *Administrative Science Quarterly, 32*(1), 106–128.

Mattera., M. (1994). Leading for tomorrow. *Registered Nurse,* 7.

Mintzberg, H. (1979). *The structuring of organizations.* Upper Saddle River, NJ: Prentice Hall.

Porter-O'Grady, T. (1999). Foreword. In B. Haag-Heitman (Ed.), *Clinical practice development using novice to expert theory* (pp. xv–xviii). Gaithersburg, MD: Aspen Publishers.

Porter-O'Grady, T., & Wilson, C. (1998). *The leadership revolution in healthcare.* Gaithersburg, MD: Aspen Publishers.

Quiñones, M. A. (1995). Pretraining context effects: Training assignment as feedback. *Journal of Applied Psychology, 80*(2), 226–238.

Robert Wood Johnson Foundation. (2009). Championing nurses in healthcare reform. Available at: www.rwjf.org/pr/product.jsp?id=38529. Accessed February 22, 2010.

Saad, L. (2008). Nurses shine, bankers slump in ethics rating. *Gallup, Inc.* Available at: www.gallup.com/poll/112264/Nurses-Shine-While-Bankers-Slump-Ethics-Ratings.aspx. Accessed February 21, 2010.

Sams, D. (1996). The development of leadership skills in clinical practice. *Nursing Times, 92*(28), 37–39.

Saunders, B. (1995). Fabled service: Ordinary acts, extraordinary outcomes. San Francisco, CA: Jossey-Bass.

Senge, P., Kleiner, A., Roberts, C., Ross, R., & Smith, B. (1994). *The fifth discipline fieldbook.* New York, NY: Doubleday Dell.

Stewart, R. (1998). *Managers and their jobs* (2nd ed.). London, England: MacMillan.

Stogdill, R. M. (1948). *Personal factors associated with leadership: A survey of the literature.* New York, NY: Free Press.

Tannenbaum, R., Weschler, I. R., & Massarik, F. (1961). *Leadership and organization: A behavioral science approach.* New York, NY: McGraw-Hill.

Tracey, J.B., Tannenbaum, S., & Kavanagh, M. (1995). Applying trained skills on the job: The importance of the work environment. *The Journal of Applied Psychology, 80*(2), 239–252.

Troyan, P. (1996). *How nurses learn about management through informal learning in the workplace* (Unpublished doctoral dissertation). Teachers College, Columbia University, New York, NY.

Waddell, D. (1992). The effects of continuing education on nursing practice: A meta-analysis. *The Journal of Continuing Education in Nursing, 23*(4), 164–168.

Yukl, G. (1994). *Leadership in organizations* (3rd ed.). Upper Saddle River, NJ: Prentice Hall.

Yukl, G., & Latham, G. (1978). Interrelationship among employee participation, individual differences, goal difficulty, goal acceptances, goal instrumentality, and performance. *Personnel Psychology, 31*(2), 305–307.

Yukl, G., & Tracey, B. (1992). Consequences of influence tactics with subordinates, peers and the boss. *Journal of Applied Psychology, 77*(4), 525–535.

# Reprint of American Nurses' Association Peer Review Guidelines—1988

## INTRODUCTION

As part of its quality assurance responsibilities, the American Nurses Association, through the Cabinet on Nursing Practice, has produced numerous documents and engaged in many activities that have influenced the development of the association's philosophy on peer review within nursing.

A system of peer review will demonstrate to the public the profession's ability to regulate itself in providing effective care. Peer review is intrinsic in self-regulation. Peer review is also one mechanism through which the profession acts to assure quality nursing care, and quality assurance is essential to the profession's advocacy of access to and recognition of nursing services.

The cost-conscious nature of today's healthcare system, challenges from other professions about nursing's role, and the current liability environment increase the importance of peer review programs. Self-regulation in nursing practice, like the practice itself, occurs in a broad social context in which there are complex dynamics, conflicting values, and finite resources. Self-regulation is a matter of conscience for the individual practitioner and the profession. To satisfy this conscience, specific knowledge, skills, and methods are required.[1]

The development of generic and specialty standards of practice, a responsibility of ANA, is an ongoing work of the association that provides a foundation for peer review. The publication *Nursing: A Social Policy Statement*[2], which describes nursing's social responsibility and the nature and scope of practice, completes the framework for building a quality assurance system with a peer review component. It is the individual nurse's responsibility to participate directly in a peer review program. This responsibility fulfills the societal contract granted through the legal license to practice and described in the Code for Nurses in terms of the nurse's ethical responsibility to maintain competence.

The association's commitment to implementing peer review was evident as early as 1973, when guidelines for peer review were prepared under the direction of the Congress for Nursing Practice. Although unpublished, the document demonstrated an understanding of nursing leaders that peer review is a necessary part of implementing the standards of practice, published in 1973. The concepts of peer review were subsequently incorporated into such publications as *Guidelines for Review of Nursing Care at the Local Level*,[3] *Quality Assurance Workbook*,[4] and *Nursing Quality Assurance Management/Learning System*.[5] In addition, ANA published a brochure, *Peer Review in Nursing Practice*,[6] in 1983 to reinforce, for nurses, other health professions, and regulatory agencies, the self-regulating nature of the nursing profession. The content from that brochure is included in this document.

## PEER REVIEW: A COMPONENT OF A QUALITY ASSURANCE SYSTEM

The American Nurses' Association believes nurses bear primary responsibility and accountability for the quality of nursing care their clients receive. Standards of nursing practice provide a means for measuring the quality of nursing care a client receives. Each nurse is responsible for interpreting and implementing the standards of nursing practice. Likewise, each nurse must participate with other nurses in the decision-making process for evaluating nursing care. This process is peer review.

Peer review implies that the nursing care delivered by a group of nurses or an individual nurse is evaluated by individuals of the same rank or standing according to established standards of practice. The goals of every agency providing nursing care should include peer review as one means of maintaining standards of nursing practice and upgrading nursing care. In every health care facility in which nurses practice and for each nurse in individual practice, provision for peer review should be an ongoing process.

### Definition of Peer Review

The generally accepted definition of *peer review* is an organized effort whereby practicing professionals review the quality and appropriateness of services ordered or performed by their professional peers. Peer review in nursing is the process by which practicing registered nurses systematically assess, monitor, and make judgments about the quality of nursing care provided by peers as measured against professional standards of practice (ANA, 1975).[7]

### Purposes and Benefits of Peer Review

Peer review's primary focus is the quality of nursing practice. However, quality, quantity, and the cost of care are closely related: what happens in one of these dimensions affects the two other dimensions. Quality control therefore includes attention to the related quantity of care (manpower utilization) and to cost control, so that patients receive only the care they need, provided at an affordable cost compatible with quality. The intent is to provide the highest quality of care at a reasonable cost. However great the external pressures for utilization and cost controls may be, the responsibility for safeguarding the quality of care is paramount.

The purposes of peer review are (a) to evaluate the quality and quantity of nursing care as it is delivered by the individual practitioner or a group of practitioners; (b) to determine the strengths and weaknesses of nursing care, taking into consideration local and institutional resources and constraints; (c) to provide evidence for use as the basis of recommendations for new or altered policies and procedures to improve nursing care; and (d) to identify those areas where practice patterns indicate more knowledge is needed.

Peer review activities are focused on the practice decisions of professional nurses to determine the appropriateness and timeliness of those decisions. The services provided as a result of practice decisions are also reviewed to determine their necessity, effectiveness, and efficiency.

Although informal peer review occurs whenever one nurse judiciously commends or critiques while assisting another in the management of care, the goals of nursing are best served by a formal process. Formal review includes, for example, the evaluation within the quality assurance system of an institution or an agency and the review necessary for third-party reimbursement for services provided by an individual or a group of nurses. An organized program makes peer review timely and objective. Peer review can occur at various levels and situations, including in primary practice, in an institution or agency, and at the local, regional, or national level.

Individuals, institutions, and the nursing profession all derive benefits from an effective peer review program. With respect to the individual, participation in the peer review process stimulates professional growth. Clinical knowledge and skills are updated. Within the institution, effective peer review points toward changes in educational and administrative patterns needed to ensure quality, and it reveals opportunities for research pertinent to the enhancement of practice. As to the profession as a whole, improved quality of care by individuals and agencies, accompanied by self-regulation of nursing practice, can only serve to strengthen nursing.

Education of nurses on the need for and value and benefits of peer review is essential. Consideration of the following benefits may encourage the individual nurse to participate in peer review and to promote its establishment in the work environment and in the professional association. Peer review—

- assures the consumer of the nurse's continued competence.
- provides an avenue for arbitration of consumer complaints, and complements risk-management programs by reducing the risk of suits.

- legally protects the competent nurse from unjust professional misconduct charges by providing documentation of the safety, competency, and expertness of the nurse's practice.
- rewards competent practice when data from peer review are incorporated into the performance appraisal and merit evaluations.
- identifies generic weaknesses in practice that can guide planning for staff development and continuing education programs and new or revised policies or procedures to improve nursing care.
- increases nurses' control over nursing practice, protecting the profession from external controls and impingement by persons outside nursing.
- helps nurses fulfill the requirement in the Code for Nurses on maintaining competency in nursing.
- provides a quality assurance mechanism and documentation for health care insurers.
- assists nurses in improving documentation, communication, and productivity.

### Interrelationship of Quality Assurance Elements

A quality assurance (QA) system is self-defining; it is simply a system that assures quality. Peer review is part of a QA system, and is best understood when placed within the context of a comprehensive QA effort. Figure 1 describes the various QA mechanisms that exist.

The three major organizational entities involved in QA in the healthcare system are institutions, professions, and regulatory agencies. Each entity uses various means to evaluate performance against standards. Institutions use audits to evaluate their business, and performance evaluations to assess their employees' work. Regulatory agencies use licensing to ensure safe, competent practice and accredit or certify institutions for quality care. Professions use certification to recognize the specialized competency of licensed individuals, and peer review to ensure the consumer of professionals' continuing competence. The six mechanisms in the diagram are complementary and may be reciprocal.

**Figure 1.  Quality assurance mechanism.**

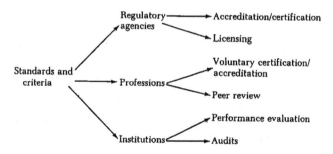

## IMPLEMENTATION OF A PEER REVIEW PROGRAM

Groups of practitioners are assisted by the profession's state and national organizational structures.

**Peer reviewers.** Peer reviewers are nurse colleagues with (a) clinical competence similar to that of the nurse seeking peer review, (b) integrity recognized by other nurses, (c) professional commitment to patients and to nursing, (d) an interest in—and knowledge about—assessing and monitoring the quality of practice, (e) demonstrated interpersonal and group work skills, and (f) demonstrated ability in both intradisciplinary and interdisciplinary collaboration. Nurse reviewers need, or must strive to develop, the judicial temperament—the capacity and the willingness to make critical decisions on the basis of evidence. A constructive approach is important in rendering judgments. Peer reviewers may be selected by appointment or by election from the total peer group.

Nurses who carry the authority and responsibility for implementing the peer review program provide a unique and vital service on behalf of patients, families, the community, their nursing colleagues, and the institution, agency, or other setting in which they work. In serving all these constituencies, they serve the profession as a whole.

**State nurses' associations.** The function of state nurses' associations is to educate the individual nurse on the peer review process. In addition, a formal mechanism, such as a standards committee, at the state level for managing appeals from consumers or nurses would be a significant quality control and service mechanism. Members of this committee could also serve as consultants to the individual nurse who is developing or participating in a peer review program.

**American Nurses' Association.** The functions of the national level of the association include (a) the enunciation of standards of practice, (b) the development of policy statements on peer review, and (c) the provision of a national system of certification for the individual nurse.

The steps in the process of peer review are the same for all nurses and all settings. The key difference lies in identifying the purpose, the peer group, and the appropriate professionally defined standards upon which to base the review. Figure 2 illustrates the basic steps in the peer review process.

### Program Guidelines

Peer review as an organized program requires written, standardized operating procedures developed and adopted by the nurses to be reviewed and by appropriate administrative bodies. The document should state (a) the intent of the peer review program in the particular setting, (b) the way the findings of peer review will be used, (c) the method of selecting reviewers, (d) the responsibilities of nurse reviewers and of management for the peer review program,

**Figure 2.    Steps in establishing a peer review program.**

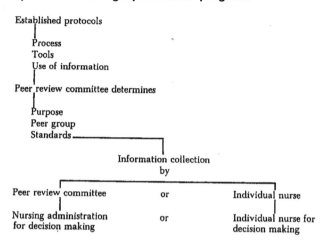

and (e) the time frame for periodic reviews or conditions under which special reviews may be conducted. In settings where self-governance or shared governance is practiced, nursing bylaws should describe the structure and functions of the peer review program.

The peer review program must provide for confidentiality with regard to patient care records and must honor the rights of the nurses being reviewed, the reviewers, the clients, the nurse administrators, and the other professionals who share responsibility for patient care.

The quality, quantity, and costs of the peer review program itself require monitoring. The operating procedures should provide for maintenance of records of the peer review process and program to permit evaluation of their efficiency and effectiveness in relation to their cost.

Since essentially the same steps are used in peer review as in other kinds of nursing practice evaluation, the seven steps of the ANA model for quality assurance in nursing are used here to organize the elements of the peer review program (ANA, 1975).[8]

1. *Identify values.* The peer group should reach consensus on which values underlying its area of practice are relevant to peer review in the specific situation. These values should be consistent with the philosophy of the nursing service department or the agency. The values should reflect the Code for Nurses, standards of practice, and other documents of the nursing profession.
2. *Identify standards and criteria.* Specific structure, process, and outcome standards relevant to the setting should be identified. Related

measurable criteria should then be elaborated as a basis for judging nurs-ing practice decisions and the quality of care resulting from the decision process. It is important for the whole group of peers, at least through representatives, to be involved in developing and adopting the standards and criteria that will be used to judge their practice.

3. *Secure measurements.* The methods for securing the descriptive or quantified data necessary for determining the degree to which stan-dards of practice and related criteria have been met should be estab-lished before their use in the peer review process. The peer group or its designated representatives should participate in the selection of data collection methods and the time frame for their use. Methods may vary from record audits to examination of reimbursement claims referred for review of nursing care.

4. *Make interpretations.* The nurse reviewers analyze the data in light of the agreed-on standards and criteria and make judgments about strengths, deficits, or other problems in quality. Further, they analyze decision points to determine that appropriate nursing care decisions were made in a timely fashion. The nursing care delivered as a result of the nursing decisions is further evaluated for its necessity, efficiency, and effectiveness, particularly when the review is associated with third-party reimbursement.

5. *Identify courses of action.* The nurse reviewers identify suitable courses of action to reward strengths, correct deficits, solve problems, and pre-vent later problems whenever possible.

6. *Choose actions.* According to the operating procedures previously defined, the nurse reviewers choose or recommend selected courses of action. If the action is to recommend, it should be directed to the most appropriate group for action. Provisions should be made for appealing the reviewers' decisions.

7. *Take action.* If empowered to do so, the nurse reviewers take the action chosen. Otherwise, they should obtain reports of follow-up on the actions recommended to others. In both cases, the results of recommended actions should be evaluated by peer review groups.

## Planning for Peer Review

The establishment of a temporary planning committee (either elected or appointed) is a starting point in providing the careful, thorough planning needed to establish a peer review program. The adoption of established profes-sional standards of practice from which guidelines for evaluating quality care may be delineated can provide a strong basis for the work of the peer groups. It would also be helpful to describe the purpose and benefit of the program and to differentiate peer review from other review situations, such as general nursing audit. The planning committee will want to consider the following:

1. Purpose and functions of the peer review committee.
2. Composition of the committee.
3. Guidelines to be used by the committee.
4. Scope and authority of the committee.
5. Policies and protocol of the committee.
6. Resource input.
7. Liability of the committee.
8. The nature of the data and the process of data collection.

The temporary planning committee will also need to consider such administrative questions as time commitment, secretarial needs, financing, frequency of meetings, and membership selection process.

It is recommended that agencies that have staff members participating on either temporary planning committees or permanent review committees should assume this cost as part of their normal operating expenses. This recommendation is based on the assumption that establishment of a peer review process will provide considerable assistance in maintaining a high standard of nursing care, thereby benefiting clients served by the agency.

The importance of involving and informing as many nurses as possible, as soon as possible, cannot be overestimated in planning for peer review. Upon completion of the ground rules, the initial planning committee should extensively publicize the concept of peer review. Open meetings should be held to give nurses the opportunity for input on the mechanics and objectives of the peer review committee. Data collected from such meetings could be taken into account when the initial planning committee outlines final objectives for the permanent committee.

After the work of the temporary committee is completed, brochures should be printed and meetings held to publicize the expected purposes, functions, and procedures of the peer review program. Meetings need to be scheduled to ensure maximum attendance by nurses affected by the peer review committee.

Members of the permanent committee or committees may be chosen according to their clinical expertise, educational background, or administrative position; by selection of at-large representatives who have earned the respect of the peer group; or by a combination of methods. The composition of the committee will be affected by the setting in which the group works.

In large agencies, each nursing department may establish its own peer review committee, with the total agency being served by a primary committee. In medium-sized agencies, one peer review committee may serve the entire agency. In small agencies or private practice, or in sparsely populated areas, the peer review committee may be made up of representatives from several health agencies and private practices.

Nurses employed in agencies with fewer than five nurses (such as a school, industry, a physician's office, or private practice) may elect their committee on a citywide or statewide basis. Private duty nurses who work in more than one facility may be reviewed by one institution on the basis of a sampling of the client population served.

## Recommendations on Structure and Procedure

### 1. *Elected Representatives*

The members should be elected by the total registered nurse group participating in the peer review process. The procedure may provide that nurses vote for their own representative (for example, a head nurse may vote for a head nurse representative, a staff nurse for a staff nurse representative) or for the total committee. Another procedure is for each party (individual or agency) involved to choose one peer and for the parties to choose one together.

The success of the committee will depend in large part on the qualifications of the members selected. This committee should be composed of practicing professional nurses who have demonstrated professional commitment (for example, by volunteering to serve on nursing committees, participating in professional organizations, and developing specific nursing expertise). It may be necessary for the membership to have expertise in a given area in order to examine a specific phenomenon successfully. Every member of the peer review committee will have an equal vote.

The committee members should have some training in group dynamics with a facilitator or consultant to prepare them for the peer review process. Areas in which development might be needed are interviewing techniques, the writing of reports, values clarification, conflict resolution, and evaluation methods.

### 2. *Committee Size*

The size of the committee will be determined by the setting, functions, and use of subcommittees. It is recommended, however, that committee membership not exceed seven persons. It has been noted that opportunities for participation by all members in groups exceeding eight are reduced and difficulty in communication among members increases. Having an odd number of committee members will prevent tie votes. In committees composed of members from several institutions, there should be at least one representative from each institution.

In order not to burden one group, it may be necessary to develop subcommittees to handle specific problems or tasks. A subcommittee could be composed of either members of the peer review committee or other persons appointed by the peer review committee and chaired by a member of the committee. As a member of the peer review committee, the subcommittee chairperson would report to the entire peer review committee at regular intervals.

### 3. *Responsibility and Status*

Peer review committees should be given the status of permanent standing committees in the organizational structure. Peer review committees should work cooperatively with other standing committees. Relationships with bodies such as the state and local nurses association, agency administration, medical staff, and certification boards and committees should be delineated and documented. This information should be available to interested parties.

Peer review committees are review bodies. The members of each peer review committee will need to determine in advance whether the results of their work can be forwarded to certification boards, nursing services, reimbursing agencies, the nurse, or others. The plan for use and distribution of information derived from peer review should be in writing and should be explained to prospective reviewers before the review process begins. Consequences of the review process such as bringing practice up to designated standards or removing practitioners from practice are the prerogative of other groups. The peer review committee, an evaluative group, is advisory to administrative or disciplinary bodies.

### 4. *Policies*

Policies need to be developed that will guide committee functioning on such issues as use of consultants, availability of review material for practitioner and client, and reliability of materials being reviewed. One of the first questions to be settled by the peer review committee is who will initiate the request for review. Will the request come from the director of nursing, individual practitioners, and/or clients?

When identifying the standards and criteria to be used in peer review, the committee will want to consider established standards of practice (such as ANA standards of practice and the Code for Nurses), state nursing practice acts, and written resources that define quality of care (professional literature).

The committee must also address questions of confidentiality and the feedback mechanism for reviewed practice. Feedback to the nurse under review is most effective when both verbal and written communication are combined. Recipients of committee feedback will, in part, be determined by who requests the review (for example, if the director of nursing requested the review, one copy would go to the director and one copy to the nurse under review). If an individual practitioner requested a review, a copy might be sent only to the individual practitioner, who then would have the option of sharing the review. The following are examples of recommended policies:

A. All involved in the peer review process should take utmost care to ensure confidentiality for the nurse under review.
B. The nurse under review is entitled to full disclosure of the committee's report on the nurse's practice.

## 5. *Procedures*

The following points refer to basic procedural considerations.

A. Review of both individual performance and group practice occurs on a regular basis at specified intervals.
B. The chairperson has the responsibility for the initial assignment of review tasks.
C. The entire committee need not review every problem. Specific problems or areas of practice may be delegated to a committee member with particular expertise in the area for initial review.
D. All assignments for initial review of the situation are made by the chairperson as soon as the request for review is received.
E. The peer review committee will determine specific data to be provided by the nurse being reviewed and will inform the nurse of his or her responsibilities for presenting material related to such activities as serving on committees, pursuing special projects, conducting research, teaching, or publishing.
F. The nurse to be reviewed should be given an opportunity for a face-to-face meeting with the peer review committee when such an encounter is appropriate to discuss problems that may have affected performance.

## 6. *Liability*

If the peer review process is operated strictly on the basis of documented facts, the legal liability of the committee is minimized.

If a nurse sued a peer review committee, the suit would probably be classified as a defamation suit. Legally, *defamation* is the injury of a person's reputation or character by statements made to a third party. There are two classes of defamation: libel and slander. Libel refers to a written statement; slander refers to an oral statement.

To avoid such suits, the peer review committee should encourage reviewers to limit comments to statements of fact that deal only with the individual's performance in a nursing capacity. Moreover, reviewers should limit comments to statements relevant to the review process. Peer reviewers are encouraged to maintain professional liability coverage that includes indemnification for claims resulting from peer review activities.

At all times, review proceedings should be carried out in accordance with established rules and principles governing the committee.

The peer review committee is entitled to examine material relevant to the reason or cause for reviewing an individual nurse or group of nurses. If such material includes patient data, every effort should be made to keep the information confidential. To avoid a lawsuit initiated by a patient, the peer review committee should conceal patient identity in records that must be reviewed.

If legal questions arise, peer review committees are urged to seek legal counsel.

### 7. Lines of Referral and Appeal

It is not realistic to assume that an effective peer review program will always arrive at decisions that are wholly acceptable to all parties involved. If the committee functions through subcommittees, the main body would be authorized to hear appeals. If any party is not in agreement with the decision rendered by the peer review committee, that party can (within a specified time) submit the reason for disagreement in writing. The nurse's right to appeal and the method for appeal should be documented and should be made available to the nurse.

An appeal may have two rationales: (a) an individual may make an appeal because the process for review was not in accordance with established rules and regulations governing the peer review committee, or (b) an individual may make an appeal because the individual questions the validity of the committee's judgment.

A nurse has a number of recourses for appeal such as the established grievance procedure or the use of a sanctioned nurse arbitrator.

## CONCLUSION

Peer review is nursing's value system made visible. This collegial process can be carried on with security in the knowledge that quantity of care, however extensive, and costs of care, however contained, lose meaning unless the quality of that care is professionally affirmed.

## REFERENCES

1. Phaneuf, Maria. *The Nursing Audit, Self-Regulation in Nursing Practice.* 2nd ed. New York: Appleton-Century-Crofts, 1976, 16.
2. American Nurses' Association. *Nursing, A Social Policy Statement.* Kansas City, Mo.: the Association, 1980.
3. American Nurses' Association. *Guidelines for Review of Nursing Care at the Local Level.* Kansas City, Mo.: the Association, 1976.
4. American Nurses' Association. *Quality Assurance Workbook.* Kansas City, Mo.: the Association, 1976.
5. American Nurses' Association and Sutherland Learning Associates. *Nursing Quality Assurance Management/Learning System.* Kansas City, Mo.: American Nurses Association, 1982.
6. American Nurses' Association. *Peer Review in Nursing Practice.* Kansas City, Mo.: the Association, 1983.
7. American Nurses' Association. *A plan for implementation of the standards of nursing practice.* Kansas City, Mo.: the Association, 1975.
8. *Ibid.*

# Just-in-Time Innovative Peer Review Strategy Improves Accuracy of Best Practice Discharge Medication Reconciliation Process

*Courtesy of East Jefferson General Hospital—Metairie, LA.*
*All rights reserved.*

During our Joint Commission survey in November, 2006, we were thrilled when the surveyors commented that the discharge medication reconciliation process we designed was "best practice." We knew from participation in the IHI 100K Lives Campaign that our next focus on the journey to medication reconciliation excellence was to improve the accuracy of the home medication list we provide to our patients at the time of discharge. In striving to improve the accuracy of the patient discharge home medication list, our team implemented many strategies, including quality management nurse audits, feedback from supervisors, numerous "hot tips," and adjustments to the computerized system. All of our efforts were met with little success until we incorporated practice-focused, just-in-time, meaningful feedback from one staff nurse to another.

*Description of our Discharge Medication Reconciliation Process*: At the time of discharge, the physician completes a medication reconciliation form and the nurse enters the medications into the electronic medical record. The nurse then prints a home medication list for the patient. Our new process calls for a nurse "peer" to check the home medication list against the original discharge medication reconciliation form for accuracy of medication names, dosages, and frequencies. The nurse "peer" then gives the primary nurse "just-in-time" feedback. Corrections are made to the list immediately and an accurate home medication list is provided to the patient.

What a difference a peer makes! Our discharge medication reconciliation accuracy rose from 56% to greater than 90% in a period of 1 year, and our improvement has been sustained for over 1 year beyond that. The essential elements of peer review that seemed to make all of the difference in dramatically improving our discharge medication reconciliation accuracy included timeliness of the feedback, a "peer" nurse from the same unit giving the feedback (as opposed to an external quality review nurse or supervisor), and the educational nature of the feedback to foster a culture of patient safety and quality (not perceived as disciplinary).

**EXAMPLE OF MORE FORMALIZED, COMPREHENSIVE, PERIODIC PEER REVIEW FOR ASSESSMENT OF NURSING PRACTICE:**

**Aligning Nursing Peer Review with Pillars of Excellence**

Our hospital uses the Five Pillars framework in setting organizational goals for excellence. In aligning our nursing peer review with institutional priorities, staff nurse groups on each unit use a template based on the pillar framework and insert the most appropriate measures for their unit under each heading. The intended effect was that the act of choosing the most relevant measures would help to reinforce each unit's high standards of care. The unexpected, but positive effects included:

1. Staff on each unit actually began to define as groups what "teamwork" and "service" really meant on their unit in terms of daily observable actions.
2. A professional development plan emerged on some units as a result of peer feedback given in the professional development measure under the heading of growth.
3. Nurses were more aware of each other's certification goals, and were able to give each other more support in achieving them.

(The Five Pillars: People, Service, Quality, Finance, and Growth, were used in this sample nursing peer review tool with permission for publication provided by the Studer Group, LLC, personal communication, October 13, 2009.)

Please find a sample of the Nursing Peer Review Tool on the following page.

## CCU Nursing
## Professional Peer Review

Peer Being Reviewed: _____
Return to: Nicole Jones (can slip under office door if off-hours) By: Friday 11/6/09

Please Note: If you feel you cannot be objective, please return this form to your supervisor. The purpose of this review is to create an environment where feedback is safe and constructive to help each other improve our clinical practice of nursing. Your comments are a very important part of this review.

**Review ONE standard in each category** (ex.-Quality, Service, etc.)

1. **Quality/Safety:** (Please check ONE standard being reviewed.)

   ☐ IV tubing labeled with date and time; and, no IVs hanging for >24 hours.
   > Circle one:     Yes     No

   ☐ Scrubs the hub with alcohol prep pad for 30 seconds before using IV.
   > Circle one:     Yes     No

   ☐ All orders are entered and accurate on 12 and/or 24 hour chart check; and all orders signed off.
   > Circle one:     Yes     No

   ☐ Lead V1 electrode in 4th intercostal space, Right sternal border.
   > Circle one     Yes     No

   ☐ ST Segment monitoring ON if appropriate for patient per CCU protocol.
   > Circle one:     Yes     No

   ☐ Medication Validation Status updated by CCU nurse when admitted to unit. (Communication order with task entered if status either "Unable to validate" or not updated.)
   > Circle one:     Updated     Not Updated

   ☐ Met standards on hand hygiene audit. (See attached audit tool.)
   > Circle one:     Met     Not Met

   ☐ Met standards on isolation audit. (See attached audit tool.)
   > Circle one:     Met     Not Met

**Example of above or more information to help peer improve his/her practice:**

_____

_____

_____

**2. People:**    (Please check ONE standard being reviewed.)

☐ Professional nursing certification (Cardiac Vascular Nurse or CCRN) (Circle the appropriate number):

    1. If certified, is mentoring one other nurse in achieving certification
    2. Is studying for certification and plans to test _____ (month/yr)
    3. Does not yet have 2 years of experience or other criteria not met
    4. No plans for certification at present, but participates in other continuing education related to cardiovascular nursing practice.

☐ Displays teamwork by:
(Circle the appropriate number):

    1. Answers call lights for patients other than your own assigned patients
    2. Offering to help a visitor/patient
    3. Offering to help other team members
    4. Responds immediately to requests for assistance
    5. Uses skilled communication to lead and direct the team during an emergency situation

**Constructive feedback to help peer achieve his/her certification goal or improve teamwork:**

_____

_____

_____

**3. Service:**    (Please check ONE standard being reviewed.)

☐ Answers all outside phone calls according to EJGH Team Member Standards:
    1. "East Jefferson General Hospital"
    2. "CCU"
    3. "This is (name)"
    4. "May I help you?"
    5. Before placing anyone on hold, asks permission and waits for a response
    6. Uses the caller's name when possible, or uses ma'am or sir.
    7. Thanks the caller for calling, holding, and/or waiting.
        Circle one:    Yes    No

☐ At the end of his/her shift, room is neat, trash is thrown away, patient is pulled up in bed, and room is stocked with essential supplies.
        Circle one:    Yes    No

**Feedback/Examples of above to help peer improve his/her practice:**

_____

_____

_____

4. **Financial:**   (Please check ONE standard being reviewed.)

☐ Charge Nurses: Staffs unit to volume of patients using new grid/other guidelines

Circle one:     1     2     3     4     5

(Rarely     Most of Time     Always)

☐ Everybody: Flexible with assignments/roles performed/floating in order to meet goals for staffing of unit and willing to accept new patients as assigned.

Circle one:     1     2     3     4     5

(Rarely     Most of Time     Always)

**Provide specific examples of above to help peer improve his/her practice:**

_____

_____

_____

5. **Growth/Technology:**   (Please check ONE standard being reviewed.)

☐ Technology: Tasks completed and addressed at end of shift.

Circle one:     Yes     No

☐ Technology: Complete/accurate charting when pulling information into INET (including accurate frequent vitals, accurate I&O, correctly pulling weights forward).

Circle one:     Yes     No

☐ Professional Development/Continuing Education:
(Check classes attended over last two years)

　　☐ Hot Cardiology Topics (Dr Dugan)
　　☐ Advanced Nursing Care of the Patient with Heart Failure (Nicole)
　　☐ Pacemaker Workshop
　　☐ Intermediate EKG
　　☐ Cardiac Vascular Nurse Board Certification Review Course
　　☐ CCRN Review Class
　　☐ Bugs and Drugs: What Nurses Should Know (Dr Blais)

    ☐ Care of the Patient undergoing an aMAZEing procedure
(Dr Brothers)
    ☐ Utilizes 12 Lead EKG Review Program on Team Talk
    ☐ Attended GNOC AACN Dinner Meeting(s)
    ☐ Attended NTI AACN National Conference
    ☐ Preceptor Workshop
    ☐ Charge Nurse Workshop
    ☐ Emotional Intelligence
    ☐ Lemons to Lemonade
    ☐ Coaching and Counseling
    ☐ Other: _____

**Provide specific example of above to help peer improve his/her
practice:**

_____

_____

**Please answer the next 2 questions on your peer:**

1. What is this team member's greatest contribution to the professional
   practice of Nursing in CCU?

2. In your opinion, what would be the area of greatest opportunity for
   improvement for this team member's clinical practice?

Signature of Peer Reviewer:

_____

Signature of Peer Being Reviewed:

_____

Date of Discussion/Feedback:

_____

# Nursing Strategic Plan

*Courtesy of Poudre Valley Hospital, Fort Collins, CO*

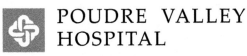

# POUDRE VALLEY HOSPITAL

POUDRE VALLEY HEALTH SYSTEM

Nursing Strategic Plan
## 2005-2008

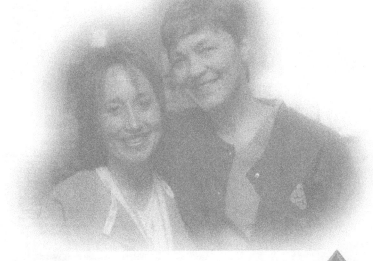

**SOLUCIENT**
TOP HOSPITALS

Poudre Valley Hospital - Fort Collins, Colorado

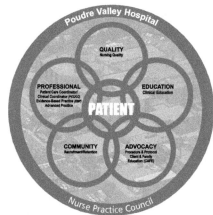

 Nursing at PVH

The Nursing **VISION:**
  Excellence in nursing.

The Nursing **MISSION:**
  To provide quality care that assists patients and families in maintaining or
  regaining health through diagnostics and interventions and learning to live
  with disabilities or dying with dignity and comfort.

The Nursing **PHILOSOPHY:**
  The nursing staff believes in a Patient/Family Centered Care Model where our
  patients are the center of quality care. Quality care is presented along the
  health continuum. Nursing care is provided through collaborative
  relationships among the patient, nursing staff and other healthcare
  providers. Nursing quality patient care is supported by a Nurse Practice
  Council comprised of Quality, Education, Advocacy, Community and
  Professional components.

PVH Nurses Support PVHS **VALUES:**
  Quality, Compassion, Confidentiality, Dignity/Respect, Equality, Integrity

# Nursing Strategic Goals 2005/2008

PVHS Strategic Goals are Supported by PVH Nursing

**STRATEGIC GOAL 1**

**Work with staff to continuously improve the culture at PVHS.**
- ✓ Maintain Magnet Status
- ✓ Evaluate Nursing Philosophy And Shared Governance Model
- ✓ Define The Purpose Of Nursing Committees In The Promotion Of Improving Clinical Care And Service
- Promote The Expansion /Development Of Nursing Research Program
- Evaluate Patient Care Model
- Implement Formal Leadership Development Curriculum
- Enhance Nurse Recruitment And Retention Plan
- Promote Nursing Certification
- Develop A Plan To Address MCR & PVH Staffing & Competence Requirements

**STRATEGIC GOAL 2**

**Strengthen and expand PVHS position as a local and regional diversified health services provider.**
- Enhance/Expand Maternal/Child Service-line
- Enhance/Expand Orthopedic Service-line
- Integrate Services With MCR
- Maintain Trauma ACS Verification And State Certification

**STRATEGIC GOAL 3**

**Differentiate and diversify the PVHS services portfolio to meet the health care needs of a growing and changing market plan.**
- Enhance/Expand Oncology Service-line
- Enhance/Expand Bariatric Service-line
- Evaluate Leading Edge Technology
  - Robotic
  - Electronic Health Record
- Assess Development of Palliative Care Services

**STRATEGIC GOAL 4**

**Build collaborative and meaningful partnerships with physicians to enhance the delivery of health care services.**
- Continue To Monitor And Improve The Process Of Patient Placement And Bed Management
- ✓ Successfully Implement The Psych ER
- Explore The Development Of A System-Wide Referral Center
- Ongoing Assessment Of Contracted Services And Programs
- Identify Criteria To Establish Behavioral Expectations For Physician Leaders

**STRATEGIC GOAL 5**

**Create a customer-focused organization with superior clinical performance and service excellence.**
- ✓ Implement Revised PVHS And Department-Based Balanced Score Cards
- ✓ Enhance Nursing Dashboard
- Maintain A State Of JCAHO Continual Readiness
- Enhance Service Excellence Program
- Successfully Implement EHR According To Established Timelines
- Identify And Implement Best Practices To Reduce "Hospital Acquired Infection Rates"
- Initiate Lemay Campus Master Plan Process And Timelines

**STRATEGIC GOAL 6**

**Sustain PVHS financial performance and strength in order to fulfill the organizations vision and goals.**
- Monitor Identified Key Financial Indicators Related To Patient Care Areas
  - Overall Expenses
  - Paid FTE
  - Cost Per Unit Of Service
  - Overtime/Double Time
  - Agency Use

**POUDRE VALLEY HOSPITAL**
POUDRE VALLEY HEALTH SYSTEM
www.pvhs.org

✓= Completed

June 2006

## POUDRE VALLEY HOSPITAL
POUDRE VALLEY HEALTH SYSTEM

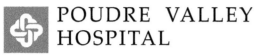

### Nurse Practice Council
Supports Magnet Forces 3, 5, 10, 12, 13
PURPOSE: To lead, coordinate and communicate the nursing activities of Poudre Valley Hospital.
CHAIR: Ryan Rohman
VICE CHAIR: Sandy Russell

### Nursing Procedure and Protocol
Supports Magnet Forces 4, 6, 12, 13
PURPOSE: To develop and recommend procedures and protocols to insure same standards of care for patient care.
CHAIR: Virginia Doty
VICE CHAIR: Cindy Black

### Evidence Based Practice
Supports Magnet Forces 6, 12, 13
PURPOSE: To utilize clinical evidence to change practice.
CHAIR: Ryan Rohman
VICE CHAIR: Gloria Bellin

### Nursing Quality
Supports Magnet Forces 6, 7, 12, 13
PURPOSE: To monitor and evaluate nursing quality activities. To identify actual or potential concerns and recommend potential solutions.
CHAIR: Marianne Strasheim
VICE CHAIR: Sharon Finch

### Clinical Education
Supports Magnet Forces 4, 11, 12, 13, 14
PURPOSE: The purpose is to coordinate and develop clinical education throughout the Poudre Valley Health System that supports innovative, high quality, and comprehensive care.
CHAIR: Linda Wilson
VICE CHAIR: Karen Moore

### Patient Care Coordinator/Clinical Coordinator
Supports Magnet Forces 12, 13
PURPOSE: A forum to support nursing leadership development through education, activities and the sharing of information.
CHAIR: Gwen Andersen
VICE CHAIR: Pam Kropp

### Retention/Recruitment
Supports Magnet Forces 4, 10, 11, 12, 13, 14
PURPOSE: To identify and recommend potential retention and recruitment activities.
CHAIR: Sara Baskin
VICE CHAIR: Laura Wining

### Client and Family Education
Supports Magnet Forces 11, 12, 13
PURPOSE: To create, develop, and implement a consistent process by which Client and Family Education is delivered throughout the organization.
CHAIR: Jeanette Fraser
VICE CHAIR: Sandy Russell

### Advanced Practice Registered Nurse
Supports Magnet Forces 8, 9
PURPOSE: Promote the advanced practice role by serving as resources and change agents to positively impact quality of care by utilizing as appropriate: evidence-based practice, education, consultation, research, quality improvement process, and/or collegial interdisciplinary relationships.
CHAIR: Jane Arndt
VICE CHAIR: Bev Moline

© June 2006
PVHS Info Design/Development

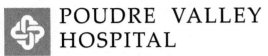

# POUDRE VALLEY HOSPITAL
POUDRE VALLEY HEALTH SYSTEM

## The Forces of Magnetism...

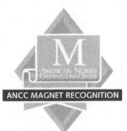

ANCC MAGNET RECOGNITION

**Force 1:** Quality of Nursing Leadership

**Force 2:** Organizational Structure

**Force 3:** Management Style

**Force 4:** Personnel Policies and Programs

**Force 5:** Professional Models of Care

**Force 6:** Quality of Care

**Force 7:** Quality Improvement

**Force 8:** Consultation and Resources

**Force 9:** Autonomy

**Force 10:** Community and the Hospital

**Force 11:** Nurses as Teachers

**Force 12:** Image of Nursing

**Force 13:** Interdisciplinary Relationships

**Force 14:** Professional Development

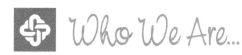

Poudre Valley Hospital (PVH) is the flagship facility of Poudre Valley Health System (PVHS). This regional hospital is located in Fort Collins, Colorado. The system consists of:

Poudre Valley Hospital
Medical Center of the Rockies
Fort Collins Family Medicine Residency
Mountain Crest Behavioral Health
Harmony Campus (MBO, Urgent Care, Imaging, One-Day Surgery)
Windsor Medical Center
Healthy Living Center
Timberline Clinic, Estes Park, CO

**PVH Overview:**
290 licensed beds
Not-for-profit
Outpatient clinics
Level II Trauma
Payer mix: 50% Medicare/Medicaid; 10% Managed Care
>2,400 employees
Average daily census: 180

**Nursing Services for 2005:**
2.66 FTE utilized in outside agency
84% RN mix
54% BSN or higher
1.5% Vacancy rate
4.6% Turnover
25.3% National Certification

**Operational Stats for 2005:**
12.49 Patient Average HPPD
3.91 LOS

Poudre Valley Health System Service Area

WYOMING   NEBRASKA
COLORADO   ★ Fort Collins

### The Culture At PVHS

**PVHS Vision:** To be a world-class health care provider.

**PVHS Mission:** To be an independent, non-profit organization and to provide innovative, high quality, comprehensive care that exceeds customer expectations.

**PVHS Values:** Quality, Compassion, Confidentiality, Dignity/Respect, Equality, Integrity

**Key Customer Requirements:** Quality Care, Friendly Staff, Prompt Service.

POUDRE VALLEY HOSPITAL
POUDRE VALLEY HEALTH SYSTEM
www.pvhs.org

# Using a Peer Review Process for Assessing Nurse Competence

*Courtesy of Decatur Memorial Hospital, Decatur, IL.*

**DECATUR MEMORIAL HOSPITAL**

**NURSING DEPARTMENT POLICY**

---

**SUBJECT:** COMPETENCY ASSESSMENT PROGRAM

**STANDARD:** MANAGEMENT OF HUMAN RESOURCES

**EFFECTIVE:** 4/92

---

**POLICY:** Nursing staff providing clinical services to patients will maintain state licensure, maintain basic competency to fulfill nursing duties, master advanced competency necessary for assigned unit, and seek learning activities for additional certification.

**IMPLEMENTATION:**

**DEFINITIONS**

**A Basic Competency**

1. An entry-level basis of knowledge and skills is required of the newly employed individual, which is established initially in the orientation process, first through a hospital-wide program and completed with a unit-specific orientation program.
2. A skills checklist is utilized to validate basic competency during orientation. It includes an introduction to the environment, knowledge of personnel issue management, information management, equipment operation, standards of

nursing care, and skills required by the position, including those specific to the age and other characteristics of the patient population being served.

### B. Advanced Competency

1. Knowledge and skills are required to perform an advanced function beyond basic nursing education, which requires additional education.
2. Nursing activities that require advanced competency validation include, but are not limited to:
   a. Sedation/analgesia administration
   b. Newborn/infant/child medication administration
   c. Neuromuscular blocker administration
   d. Oxytocin administration
   e. Internal fetal monitor lead application
   f. Pediatric code pink
   g. Pulmonary artery pressure monitoring
   h. Pulmonary artery catheter removal
   i. Intravenous chemotherapy administration
   j. Advanced IV administration of cardiovascular agents
   k. Code Blue

**NOTE:** A unit-specific advanced competency assessment for additional nursing activities will be determined by the director of the unit and advanced practice staff.

### C. Certification/Licensure

1. The process concerned with external validation of competency achieved via a recognized licensing or accrediting body, professional association, or higher learning institution.
2. State licensure is required for nursing personnel in conjunction with the Illinois Nursing Act of 1987. Documentation will be kept in the employee file. Nurses may not practice without proof of licensure.
3. Additional certification and/or licensing is encouraged but not required.

## COMPETENCY PROCESS

A. Evaluation of competence will begin in the employment process and continue on a regular basis throughout the employment period.
B. Competence is validated by designated persons during nursing orientation and with a preceptor. Documentation will be kept in the employee personnel file.
C. Advanced competency may require a formal educational experience initially and validated through a process that includes a criterion-based assessment of knowledge and application via skill demonstration and/or written examination. A nurse proficient in that particular skill evaluates

and validates advanced competency. Documentation will be kept in the employee personnel file.

D. Ongoing Competency Evaluation
1. Competencies will be revalidated <u>at least annually</u> as a part of the evaluation process.
2. The method for evaluation of competencies will be the use of peer review process as governed by the Clinical Practice Committee. Frequency of evaluation of competencies will be determined by each unit director with assistance from the advanced practice staff and/or the Education Department and Clinical Practice Committee based on the following:
    a. Procedures that are problem prone or high risk
    b. High-volume procedures
    c. External standards/internal standards
    d. Specific specialty recommendation
    e. Quality improvement
3. Variances from acceptable performance standards may trigger competence assessment activities for an individual or a group of individuals at any time.

E. The Human Resources Department will report competency assessment to the Board of Directors annually.

F. Code Blue competency requires that the registered nurse (RN) be competent in:
    a. Cardiopulmonary resuscitation
    b. Basic arrhythmia
    c. Advanced cardiac life support (ACLS)
    d. Advanced IV cardiac medications and complete a skill demonstration and written examination

Only Code Blue competent RNs will be allowed to:
    a. Initiate standard orders for arrhythmia
    b. Act as team leader in Code Blue

G. Only RNs with advanced competency in sedation analgesia may administer sedation analgesia. The RN must be competent in basic arrhythmia interpretation and ACLS.

**APPLICABLE TO:**     All Nursing Departments

**APPROVED BY:**

_____

Vice President, Chief Nurse Executive

Revised: 5/98, 11/98, 4/01, 1/08, 10/08

Peer Review Process

Medication Reconciliation

Instructions for Use of Tool

1.  Knows what to do at admission if patients do not know meds:

Have them tell you what steps that they take to get the med list from other resources if the patient is a poor historian or unable to communicate. Hopefully they mention the physician's office, family members, pharmacies, etc. If nothing else, they should tell you that they document the reason for an incomplete med list.

2.  Knows the process for medical records for nursing home discharges:

Make sure they tell you that for nursing homes, there needs to be a copy sent to the nursing home and a copy retained with the permanent record. Often, people forget to leave a copy with the permanent record. Make sure the med list is faxed to the nursing home ahead of time and then confirmed during verbal report that they received it, and everything is clear and makes sense. It is best if the person is observed in doing the process so that you can know that they are doing it appropriately.

3.  Knows the process for medical records for discharges to home:

Make sure that the patient gets a copy of the discharge meds as well as having a copy in the chart for the permanent record. Make sure to tell the patient to keep a list of meds in their purse or wallet and to show the list to their physician offices. They need to update the list with every change in regimen. Remind them to bring the list to the hospital anytime they are here no matter what reason. Make sure to add prescriptions to the electronic list and update every field even if things are being kept the same. Watch the person doing a real discharge to make sure they are doing the process appropriately.

4.  Takes appropriate action at admission with unreconciled medications:

Make sure that they know to check with the physician about any home meds that are not addressed on the medical records form and not documented in progress notes as being stopped intentionally. If there is an obvious reason not documented by the physician, the nurse needs to make a note in the chart.

5.  Informs patients of reasons for changes to their usual routine medication regimen:

Watch the person doing some patient education about home meds. Also, ask a couple of patients that the person has admitted if they were given information about their medication regimen for their hospital stay.

*Peer Competency Example—Medication Reconciliation*

Name/Date: _____

Peer Review Process for RN's

Medication Reconciliation

April–June 2009

| Skill | Criteria | (2/3) Met Initial/ Date | *Not Met | N/A | Comments *Any item "not met" must be addressed with a comment. |
|---|---|---|---|---|---|
| Knows what to do at admission if patient does not know meds | Based on interview | | | | |
| Knows the process for medical records for nursing home discharges | Based on interview and demonstration | | | | |
| Knows the process for medical records for discharges to home | Based on interview and demonstration | | | | |
| Takes appropriate action at admission with unreconciled medications | Based on interview by reviewer and demonstration | | | | |
| Informs patient of reasons for changes to their usual routine medication regimen | Based on interview of nurse and patients, and on demonstration | | | | |

**Please write legibly**    1. Reviewer/Initial: _____

2. Reviewer/Initial: _____

3. Reviewer/Initial: _____

Peer Review Process

Fall Prevention

Instructions for Use of Tool

1. <u>Knows how to identify patients at risk for falls:</u>

   Ask them to name things that contribute to patient falls (new environment, medications, having to use the bathroom in a hurry, etc.). Ask them to show you how they document a fall risk assessment in the charting system.

2. <u>Initiates fall risk interventions per protocol if indicated:</u>

   Find out what patients your person that you are reviewing is caring for and review three of those charts for appropriate documentation of fall risk interventions depending on risk level as identified in the patient's fall risk assessment.

3. <u>Evidence is found in patient room that supports what is documented in patient record:</u>

   Look at fall risk assessment and intervention charting on one or two of their patients and then walk to the room and see if the interventions are actually in place.

4. <u>Knows how to provide continuity of care for fall risk patients from department to department:</u>

   Ask them to tell you what they provide in report to the receiving nurses when a patient is a fall risk. What supplies are transferred with the patient? How do they make sure that the next department or ancillary department (radiology, interventional, transportation, etc.) knows that the patient is a fall risk.

5. <u>Provides education to patient and family on fall risk prevention:</u>

   They are able to state ways that they educate the patient and family in order to gain their support on helping to prevent falls. Do they chart that they provide this education?

Name/Date: _____

Peer Review Process

Fall Prevention

March 2009

| Skill | Criteria | (2/3) Met Initial/ Date | *Not Met | N/A | Comments *Any item "not met" must be addressed with a comment. |
|---|---|---|---|---|---|
| Knows how to identify patients at risk for falls | Based on review of documentation of three charts | | | | |
| Initiates fall risk interventions per protocol if indicated | Based on interview and demonstration | | | | |
| Evidence is found in patient room that supports what is documented in patient record | Based on interview | | | | |
| Knows how to provide continuity of care for fall risk patients from department to department | Based on interview by reviewer | | | | |
| Provides education to patient and family on fall risk prevention | Based on chart reviews and examination of patient rooms | | | | |

**Please write legibly**

1. Reviewer/Initial: _____

2. Reviewer/Initial: _____

3. Reviewer/Initial: _____

# Texas Board of Nursing: Peer Review

*Available at http://www.bon.state.tx.us/practice/faq-peerreview.html.
Accessed October 22, 2009.*

**FAQs—NURSING PEER REVIEW**

**General Peer Review Information**

**(1) What is Peer Review? [Nursing Peer Review (NPR) §303.001(5)]**

Peer review is the evaluation of nursing services, the qualifications of a nurse, the quality of patient care rendered by nurses, the merits of a complaint concerning a nurse or nursing care, and a determination or recommendation regarding a complaint including:

a. the evaluation of the accuracy of a nursing assessment and observation and the appropriateness and quality of the care rendered by a nurse;

b. a report made to a nursing peer review committee concerning an activity under the committee's review authority;

c. a report made by a nursing peer review committee to another committee or to the Board as permitted or required by law; and

d. implementation of a duty of a nursing peer review committee by a member, an agent, or an employee of the committee.

A Peer Review Committee may review the nursing practice of a LVN, RN, or APN (RN with advanced practice authorization).

There are two kinds of nursing peer review:

1. **Incident-based (IBPR)**, in which case peer review is initiated by a facility, association, school, agency, or any other setting that utilizes the services of nurses; or

2. **Safe Harbor (SHPR)**, which may be initiated by a LVN, RN, or APN prior to accepting an assignment or engaging in requested

191

conduct that the nurse believes would place patients at risk of harm, thus potentially causing the nurse to violate his/her duty to the patient(s). Invoking safe harbor in accordance with rule 217.20 protects the nurse from licensure action by the BON as well as from retaliatory action by the employer.

See revised rules 217.19 (Incident-Based Nursing Peer Review and Whistleblower Protections) and 217.20 (Safe Harbor Peer Review and Whistleblower Protections) (http://www.bon.state.tx.us/nursinglaw/rr.html)

**(2) What is a nursing peer review committee? [NPR §303.001(4); 22TAC 217.19(a)(14), 217.20(a)(14)]**

It is a committee established under the authority of the governing body of a national, state, or local nursing association; a school of nursing; the nursing staff of a hospital, health science center, nursing home, home health agency, temporary nursing service, or other healthcare facility; or state agency or political subdivision for the purpose of conducting nursing peer review. The nursing peer review process is one of fact-finding, analysis, and study of events by nurses in a climate of collegial problem solving focused on obtaining all relevant information about an event.

**(3) Who must have a peer review plan? [NPR §303.0015 ]**

Any person or entity that employs, hires, or contracts for the services of 10 or more nurses (RNs, LVNs or any combination thereof) must have a Peer Review Plan; however, peer review of RNs is not mandatory if the facility employs less than 5 RNs. A person or entity required to have nursing peer review may contract with another entity to conduct nursing peer review.

**(4) What is the Peer Review committee's composition? (NPR §303.003)**

NPR law, Section 303.003(a) requires that a Nursing Peer Review Committee that conducts a review that involves the practice of registered nurses and licensed vocational nurses must have registered nurses and licensed vocational nurses as 3/4 of its members;

NPR Law Section 303.003 (b) requires that a Nursing Peer Review Committee that conducts a review that involves the practice of licensed vocational nurses must:

a. to the extent feasible, include licensed vocational nurses as members; and

b. have only registered nurses and licensed vocational nurses as voting members.

Section 303.003(c) requires that a Nursing Peer Review Committee that conducts a peer review that involves the practice of professional nursing (including a RN with advanced practice authorization) must:

a. have registered nurses as 2/3 of its members;
b. have only registered nurses as voting members; and
c. where feasible, have at least one nurse with a working familiarity of the area of nursing practice of the nurse being reviewed. If APN practice is reviewed, preferably have an APN with authorization in the same role and specialty on peer review or advising peer review.

In addition, rule 217.19(d)(3)(B) and rule 217.20(h)(2)(B)-(C) exclude from membership or attendance at the Peer Review Committee hearing any person(s) with administrative authority for personnel decisions directly relating to the nurse. A person with administrative authority over the nurse may only appear as a fact witness.

**(5) What part of the Peer Review process is confidential? [NPA §303.006-.007; §303.0075, rule 217.19(h), §217.20(j)]**

All proceedings of the nursing Peer Review committee are confidential and all communications made to the committee are privileged. All information made confidential is not subject to subpoena or discovery in any civil matter, is not admissible as evidence in any judicial or administrative proceeding, and may not be introduced into evidence in a nursing liability suit arising out of the provision of, or failure to provide, nursing services. SB993 (80th Legis Session (2007)) added §303.0075 that addresses protection of information shared between the peer review committee and a patient safety committee under §301.457(g).

**(6) To whom may the SHPR Committee disclose privileged information (NPR §303.007)?**

Upon written request, the committee shall disclose written or oral communications and the records and proceedings of the committee to:

1. the State Board of registration or licensure of any state; or
2. a law enforcement authority investigating a criminal matter.

A nursing peer review committee may disclose written or oral communications made to the committee and the records and proceedings of the committee to:

1. a licensing agency of any state;
2. a law enforcement agency investigating a criminal matter;

3. the association, school, agency, facility, or other organization under whose authority the committee is established (i.e., employer);
4. another nursing peer review committee;
5. a peer assistance program approved by the board under Chapter 457, Health and Safety Code;
6. an appropriate state or federal agency, or accrediting organization that accredits [a] healthcare facility or school of nursing or surveys a facility for quality of care; or
7. a person engaged in bona fide research, if all information that identifies a specific individual is deleted.

**(7) Is it acceptable to use an informal work group of the peer review committee for either incident-based or safe harbor peer review? Do the same time lines apply for conducting the review when using an informal work group of the peer review committee? [rule 217.19(e) or 217.20(k)]**

Yes, any entity conducting peer review may choose to use a smaller work group of the peer review committee for either incident-based or safe-harbor peer review. A nurse involved as the primary party in peer review does not waive any due process rights by agreeing to work with an informal work group, including the right to have an issue heard by the entire peer review committee. See rule 217.19(e) or 217.20(k) for specific requirements when using a smaller work group of the peer review committee. Also review rule 217.16 Minor Incidents regarding use of a smaller work group of the nursing peer review committee.

**(8) Can we just use the BON Nursing Peer Review statutes and rules as our facility/agency policies and procedures on Nursing Peer Review?**

No, many other details must be included in peer review policies and procedures in order to have an operational peer review committee structure. As the BON does not regulate practice settings of any kind, the Board does not have authority to prescribe every aspect of peer review at the facility or employer level.

Examples of issues that must be addressed in facility policies include (but are not limited to):

- How many nurses (LVN and RN) make up the nursing peer review committee (PRC)?
- How long does a nurse serve on the nursing peer review committee?
- How is the facility's legal counsel involved in nursing peer review, and how does the facility assure "parity of counsel?"

- How will documents of the nursing PRC and the Patient Safety Committee be marked so that the origin of any "shared" documents can be determined in order to comply with NPR §303.0075(c).
- Requirements specified in both rules when use an Informal Workgroup of Peer Review Committee.

Entities desiring to establish or substantially revise their nursing peer review policies and procedures may find it helpful to contact professional organizations that represent nurses or healthcare settings. Such organizations may have developed generic policies, forms, etc., on nursing peer review for the benefit of their membership, and may have such information available for sale to the public.

**(9) What records should a peer review committee chairperson maintain, and for how long? What records should the PRC chairperson send to the board when subpoenaed by the BON to send "all nursing peer review records related to "Jane Doe RN?"**

The NPR statute does not specify requirements related to records retention of peer review proceedings, nor has the board established any time frame by rule. With the ability to scan and save documents in a digital format, the BON would encourage facilities and employers to consider this permanent method of archiving peer review documents. There is no statute of limitations on when nursing violations can be reported to the BON, including alleged violations of the nurse's due process rights in relation to a nursing peer review proceeding. Therefore, if permanent archiving is not possible, then the longest retention period possible is encouraged.

The PRC chair is responsible for maintaining all records pertaining to a peer review proceeding, including but not limited to, copies of facility policies in effect at the time of the PRC proceeding;, identities of the specific nurses who were members of the PRC and designation of their licensure and area of practice, relevant documents–such as staffing schedules, assignment sheets, staffing plans/policies, medical record numbers and dates of the involved patients, copies of the notice letter sent to the nurse and proof that the nurse received it or that the letter was returned, SHPR forms signed by the nurse and applicable staff throughout the stages of the peer review process, and documents showing the peer review committee's determination. All documents of this nature related to the peer review proceeding should be included when a subpoena of "all peer review documents" is received from the BON.

**(10) What whistleblower protections does a nurse have if he/she reports a facility, agency, school or other entity that provides healthcare services, or a physician or other licensed practitioner for endangering patients/clients or engaging in unethical or illegal conduct? [NPA§ 301.4025, §301.413]**

The above listed sections of the NPA Chapter 301, and rules 217.19(m) and 217.20(l) address protections a nurse has when reporting unsafe practices of practitioners other than nurses (such as physicians, dentists, etc.) or entities (such as hospitals, nursing homes, home health agencies, etc.). The BON does not regulate practitioners who are not nurses, or facilities, agencies, or other entities that utilize the services of nurses. Thus, reports regarding other practitioners or entities should be reported to the appropriate licensing or regulatory agency. Should a nurse experience or be threatened with retaliatory measures for reporting unsafe conditions or practitioners, staff [should] advise the nurse to seek his/her own legal counsel for guidance.

### Incident-Based Nursing Peer Review

**(1) What "due process" rights must the peer review committee provide to the nurse undergoing Incident-Based Peer Review (IBPR)? [rules 217.19(d)]**

Review of NPR Chapter 303 in its entirety is recommended, as compliance with various sections of this chapter is necessary to assure compliance with "due process" and "good faith" peer review requirements. Rule 217.19(d) delineates specific requirements for minimum due process during IBPR. Committee membership and voting requirements are described in NPR §303.003(a)-(d); §303.0015, and §217.19(c) and (d)(3)(B).

The nurse being peer reviewed must receive notification of the peer review process as well as other components that are part of the nurse's minimum due process rights under §217.19(d) including:

- that his/her practice is being evaluated by the nursing peer review committee,
- that the peer review committee will meet on a specified date not less than 21, but not more than 45 calendar days from the date of notice,
- a copy of the peer review plan, policies, and procedures.
- the notice must include:
  - a description of the event(s) to be evaluated in enough detail to inform the nurse of the incident, circumstances and conduct, and should include date(s), time(s), location(s), and individual(s) involved. Any patient or client information shall be identified by

initials or number to protect confidentiality, but the nurse shall be provided the name of the patient.
- ○ the name, address and telephone number of the contact person to receive the nurse's response (typically the peer review chairperson).
- the nurse is provided the opportunity to review, in person or by attorney, at least 15 calendar days prior to appearing before the committee, documents concerning the event under review.
- the nurse is provided the opportunity to appear before the committee, make a verbal statement, ask questions and respond to questions of the committee, and provide a written statement regarding the event under review.
- the nurse shall have the opportunity to:
  - ○ call witnesses, question witnesses, and be present when testimony or evidence is being presented;
  - ○ be provided copies of the witness list and written testimony or evidence at least 48 hours in advance of the proceeding;
  - ○ make an opening statement to the committee;
  - ○ ask questions of the committee and respond to questions of the committee; and
  - ○ make a closing statement to the committee after all evidence is presented.
- the committee must complete its evaluation within 14 calendar days from the date of the peer review hearing.
- within 10 calendar days of completion of the peer review hearing, the peer review committee must notify the nurse in writing of its determination.
- the nurse shall be given an opportunity, within 10 calendar days, to provide a written rebuttal to the committee's findings which shall become a permanent part of the peer review records.

**(2) May the employer take disciplinary action prior to conducting Incident-Based Peer Review? [NPA 301.405(e)]**

Employment and licensure issues are separate. An employer may take disciplinary action before review by the peer review committee is conducted, as peer review cannot determine issues related to employment. The role of peer review is to determine if licensure violations have occurred and, if so, if the violations require reporting to the board. If a report to the BON is already required under 301.405(c), then the role of the peer review committee is to investigate whether external factors impacted the error or situation, and to report their findings to a patient safety committee if they determine there were external factors that mitigate or aggravate the circumstances impacting the nurse's actions.

**(3) Does an employer have to report to the Board if they terminate a nurse, or make an agency nurse a "do-not-return," for practice-related errors? [Section 301.405 (b)]**

If an employer terminates a nurse for non-practice-related reasons (such as too many absences, or non-patient-related misconduct) this is an employment, not licensure, issue and is not board-reportable.

If an employer terminates a nurse (voluntarily or involuntarily), suspends for seven (7) or more days, or takes other substantive disciplinary action against a nurse or substantially equivalent action against an agency nurse for nursing practice errors/concerns, the employer must report to the Board (BON) in writing:

1. the identity of the nurse;
2. the conduct subject to reporting that resulted in the termination, suspension, or other substantive disciplinary action or substantially equivalent action; and
3. any additional information the board requires.

**(4) Does IBPR Committee have to meet if the nurse voluntarily resigns or is involuntarily terminated for practice related reasons? Does the nurse have due process rights under peer review if a report to the BON is already mandatory under NPA §301.405(b) or §301.402(b)? [NPA §301.405(c) and rule 217.19(f)(1)]**

SB993 (80th Legis. Session, 2007) amended NPA ( TOC) §301.405(c) requiring that even if a mandatory report by the employer has been, or will be, made to the BON under §301.405(b), the peer review committee must still meet to determine if external factors beyond the nurse's control impacted the nurse's deficiency in care. If the peer review committee believes external factors were involved in the incident (whether or not the nurse is being reported to the BON) the committee is now required to also report the issue to the entity's patient safety committee, or to the CNO/nurse administrator if there is no patient safety committee.

Because the nursing peer review committee is reviewing the incident solely to determine existence of external factors, due process rights of incident-based peer review do not apply. In addition, a peer review committee cannot make a determination that would negate the duty of the employer to report the nurse under §301.405(b) or of the CNO/nurse administrator to report the nurse under §301.402(b).

**(5) Must the recommendations made by the IBPR Committee be followed by the employer?**

The nursing peer review committee does not have authority to make employment or disciplinary decisions. The employer must make their own decision about appropriate disciplinary actions; however, the employer may choose to utilize the decisions of the peer review committee in determining what action they wish to take with regard to the nurse's employment. In addition, an employer may not prohibit a peer review committee from filing a report to the BON if the PRC has determined in good faith that a nurse's practice must be reported to the Board in compliance with §301.403, rule 217.11(1)(K), and rule 217.19.

**(6) What is a Minor Incident? [NPA301.419(a), rule §217.16(b)]**

A "minor incident" is defined by Texas Occupations Code (Nursing Practice Act) §301.419(a) as "conduct that does not indicate that the continuing practice of nursing by an affected nurse poses a risk of harm to the client or other person."

**(7) Are there Exclusions to What Can Be Considered a Minor Incident? [rule 217.16]**

Yes. Rule 217.16(c) defines 3 types of circumstances in which the conduct cannot be considered a minor incident:

1. Any error that contributed to a patient's death;
2. Criminal conduct defined in NPA 301.4535; or
3. A serious violation of the board's Unprofessional Conduct rule 217.12 involving intentional or unethical conduct such as fraud, theft, patient abuse or patient exploitation.

**(8) What are the criteria for determining if Minor Incidents are Board reportable?**

Rule 217.16(d) establishes when a minor incident is or is not board-reportable: (d) Criteria for Determining if Minor Incident is Board-Reportable.

1. A nurse involved in a minor incident need not be reported to the Board unless the conduct:
   a. creates a significant risk of physical, emotional, or financial harm to the client;
   b. indicates the nurse lacks a conscientious approach to or accountability for his/her practice;
   c. indicates the nurse lacks the knowledge and competencies to make appropriate clinical judgments and such knowledge and competencies cannot be easily remediated; or

        d. indicates a pattern of multiple minor incidents demonstrating that the nurse's continued practice would pose a risk of harm to clients or others.

    2. Evaluation of Multiple Incidents.

        a. Evaluation of Conduct. In evaluating whether multiple incidents constitute grounds for reporting, it is the responsibility of the nurse manager or supervisor, or peer review committee to determine if the minor incidents indicate a pattern of practice that demonstrates the nurse's continued practice poses a risk and should be reported.

        b. Evaluation of Multiple Incidents. In practice settings with nursing peer review, the nurse shall be reported to peer review if a nurse commits **five minor incidents within a 12-month period.** In practice settings with no nursing peer review, the nurse who commits five minor incidents within a 12 month period shall be reported to the Board.

**(9) What is the Peer Review committee required to report? [NPA §301.401, 301.403, & rule 217.11, rule 217.12, rule 217.16]**

A peer review committee is required to make a report to the Board if they believe in good faith that a nurse has engaged in conduct subject to reporting as defined under the Nursing Practice Act (NPA), §301.401(1). This nearly always involves one or more suspected violations of Rules 217.11, Standards of Nursing Practice, or 217.12, Unprofessional Conduct, or may fail to meet the criteria for consideration as a minor incident [217.16(c) Exclusions, or 217.16(d) discussed above].

If a Peer Review committee finds that a nurse engaged in conduct that is subject to reporting, the committee must file a signed, written report to the BON that includes:

    1. the identity of the nurse;

    2. a description of any corrective action that was taken;

    3. a recommendation whether the Board should take formal disciplinary action against the nurse and the basis for the recommendation;

    4. a description of the conduct subject to reporting [defined under 301.401(1)];

    5. the extent to which any deficiency in care provided by the nurse was the result of a factor beyond the nurse's control; and

    6. any additional information the board requires.

\* Failure to classify an event appropriately in order to avoid reporting the nurse to the BON may result in action against the nurse or nurses on the peer review committee responsible for reporting, and/or the CNO who failed to report to the board under his/her duty as a nurse in compliance with NPA §301.402.

**(10) If a nurse's practice is suspected of being impaired secondary to chemical dependency, drug or alcohol abuse, substance abuse/ misuse, "intemperate use,"mental illness, or diminished mental capacity, must Peer Review be conducted and a report filed with the Board? [NPA §301.410 & Rule 217.19(g)]**

It depends. If there is no evidence of nursing practice violations, a nurse may be reported to either the BON or to a peer assistance program [rule 217.19(g)(1)].

However, if, during the course of an incident-based peer review process, there is evidence of nursing practice violations in conjunction with evidence of impaired nursing practice, the incident-based peer review process must be suspended, and the nurse reported to the board in accordance with NPA (TOC) §301.410(b) (relating to a required report to the board when practice errors exist with suspected or known impairment of the nurse). The BON will determine in such cases whether or not the nurse is eligible to take part in a peer assistance program.

The IBPR committee may need to re-convene for the sole purpose of determining whether or not external factors contributed to the incident(s) that lead to peer review. Remember that because the nurse's practice is not being reviewed (only the surrounding factors), due process rights for the nurse do not apply.

**(11) Who conducts Peer Review for a temporary or contract employee? (NPR §303.004)**

The nurse who works through a temporary agency or contractor may be subject to Peer Review by either the facility where services are provided, the compensating agency, or both. For purposes of exchange of information, the Peer Review committee reviewing the conduct is considered as established under the authority of both so that confidentiality requirements of peer review are enforceable against any nurse involved in the investigation or peer review proceeding. The two entities may choose to have a contract with respect to which entity will conduct Peer Review of the nurse.

## Safe Harbor Peer Review

**(1) What is Safe Harbor? [NPR §303.005(b) and (e); Rule 217.19(a)(15), Rule 217.20(a)(15)]**

Safe Harbor is a nursing peer review process that a nurse may initiate when asked to engage in an assignment or conduct that the nurse believes in good faith would potentially result in a violation of Board Statutes or Rules. When properly invoked, safe harbor protects a nurse from employer retaliation and from licensure sanction by the BON. Safe Harbor must be invoked prior to engaging in the conduct or assignment for which peer review is requested, and may be invoked at any time during the work period when the initial assignment changes.

Examples of Safe Harbor situations include clinical assignments related to staffing and/or acuity of patients where the nurse believes patient harm may result {217.11(1)(B) and (T)}, and can involve a request to engage in unprofessional or illegal conduct, such as falsifying medical record documents. The latter is an example of a situation where a prudent nurse would refuse to engage in the conduct requested. {NPA §301.352(a-1), rule 217.20(g)(1)(B)}

Safe Harbor also allows for a nurse to request that a determination be made on the medical reasonableness of a physician's order [NPR 303.005(e)]. {Note: There is now a separate form on the BON web page that can be used for this process.}

**(2) What protections of a nurse's license are applicable under Safe Harbor? [NPA §301.352, §301.413; NPR §303.005(c), (d), and (h)]**

A nurse who in good faith requests Safe Harbor peer review:

1. may not be disciplined or discriminated against for making the request;
2. may engage in the requested conduct pending the peer review;
3. is not subject to the reporting requirement under Subchapter I, Chapter 301; and
4. may not be disciplined by the board for engaging in that conduct while the peer review is pending.

**(3) Where do I send my Safe Harbor request? Do I Fax it to the Board of Nursing?**

Please <u>DO NOT</u> mail or fax your request for Safe Harbor Nursing Peer Review to the Board of Nursing. The BON cannot conduct Peer Review—this must be done through the facility or agency where the assignment was made to you. Please review the following questions, as well as the instructions on the Comprehensive Request for Safe Harbor form (located under the Nursing Practice link, and then under Nursing Peer Review on the BON web page http://www.bon.state.tx.us/practice/pdfs/SHPR-CompRequest.pdf

**(4) How does a nurse invoke these protections? [Rule 217.20(d)]**

To activate Safe Harbor protections, the nurse must:

1. At the time the nurse is requested to engage in the activity, notify the supervisor making the assignment in writing that the nurse is invoking Safe Harbor. The nurse may use the BON's Quick Request Form (or any document that contains the minimum information required by rule), or may use any other means of recording the initial request for safe harbor in writing with at least the minimum information required under §217.20(d)(3)(i)-(v):

   a. The nurses(s) name(s) making the safe harbor request and his/her signature(s);

   b. The date and time of the request;

   c. The location of where the conduct or assignment is to be completed;

   d. The name of the person requesting the conduct or making the assignment; and

   e. A brief explanation of why safe harbor is being requested.

This written Quick Request for safe harbor may be brief, but before leaving at the end of the work period, the nurse must submit a written Comprehensive Request (detailed account) of his/her request for safe harbor. Additional supporting documents may still be supplied at a later date. Quick Request and Comprehensive Request for Safe Harbor forms are available on the BON web site under the Nursing Practice link. There is also a separate form for requesting a determination regarding the Medical Reasonableness of a Physician's Order. All of these BON forms are optional and do not have to be utilized by the nurse making a written request for Safe Harbor.

**(5) If a nurse invokes Safe Harbor, and the Supervisor subsequently is able to remedy the situation that caused the nurse to invoke Safe Harbor (such as obtaining more staff), is the nurse's request for Safe Harbor invalid? Does the nurse have to withdraw his/her request for a nursing peer review committee to evaluate the nurse's request?**

The nurse's request for Safe Harbor Peer Review does not become invalid and the nurse does not have to withdraw his/her request for Safe Harbor just because a supervisor is able to respond with adequate staff, equipment or whatever else was at issue with the original requested assignment. It is the nurse's choice whether or not he/she wishes to still have a nursing peer review of the situation. {See the Comprehensive Request for Safe Harbor form http://www.bon.state.tx.us/practice/pdfs/SHPR-CompRequest.pdf

under Section I The Nurse's Request, #10 Nurse's Decision to Sustain or Withdraw Request for Safe Harbor Peer Review}

## (6) When Can a Nurse Invoke Safe Harbor and Refuse the Assignment? [NPA (TOC) §301.352, rule 217.20(g)]

The NPA, section 301.352 permits a nurse to refuse an assignment when the nurse believes in good faith that the requested conduct or assignment could constitute grounds for reporting the nurse to the board under NPA 301.401(1), could constitute a minor incident, or could constitute another violation of the board statutes or rules. Situations involving potential risk of harm to patients or the public are referred to as "violating the nurse's duty to the patient" because all nurses have a duty under rule 217.11(1)(B) to maintain a safe environment for patients/clients and others for whom the nurse is responsible. Safe Harbor enables a nurse in most circumstances to accept the assignment, thus allowing the nurse to protect his/her nursing license from board sanctions while at the same time delivering the best care possible to a patient(s).

Patients are better off with the nurse than without the nurse in the vast majority of cases; however, rule 217.20(g) clarifies that a nurse may engage in an assignment or requested conduct pending peer review determination unless the requested assignment or conduct is one that:

1. constitutes a criminal act
2. constitutes unprofessional conduct, or
3. the nurse lacks the basic knowledge, skills, and abilities necessary to deliver nursing care that is safe and that meets the minimum standards of care to such an extent that accepting the assignment would expose one or more patients to an unjustifiable risk of harm.

A request to falsify a patient record is an example of conduct that a nurse should refuse to engage in while awaiting a peer review committee determination, since there is no legal or factual basis that would support a nurse falsifying a patient record. A request to accept an assignment when a nurse believes the nurse staffing levels are unsafe would be conduct a nurse normally would engage in pending peer review's determination since the supervisor normally would have some reasonable legal or factual basis to support her/his belief that the requested assignment does not violate a nurse's duty to a patient, even if peer review ultimately determines otherwise.

While §217.11(1)(B) establishes the nurse's duty to maintain patient safety, standard §217.11(1)(T) requires each nurse to "accept only those nursing assignments that take into consideration client safety and that are commensurate with the nurse's educational preparation, experience, knowledge, and physical and emotional ability." It is also impossible in the rule-writing process to anticipate every possible situation a nurse might face in every practice setting, and where a nurse may believe in good faith that his/her duty to one or more patients is in greater jeopardy to accept the assignment than to refuse it. The BON urges each nurse to consider the duty to the patient(s) as the highest priority in mak[ing] any determination to accept or refuse an assignment or requested conduct. The ability to invoke Safe Harbor protections and to have a nursing peer review committee evaluate the requested assignment are the same whether the nurse accepts or refuses the assignment.

Note that rule 217.20(g)(2) now requires the nurse and supervisor to collaborate in an effort to identify an assignment that "is within the nurse's scope and enhances the delivery of safe patient care." This is based on the premise that in any staffing crisis, the patients are almost always better off with the nurse, than without the nurse. A collaborative effort with patient safety as the focus will require the nurse and supervisor to set aside any personal animosity and to explore additional options that are safer for both the patient(s) and the nurse(s).

### (7) Does Safe Harbor Protect a Nurse from Civil or Criminal Liability? [NPR §303.005(h), 217.20(e)(2) & (3)]

No. Safe Harbor has no effect on a nurse's civil or criminal liability for his/her nursing practice. The BON does not have any authority over civil or criminal liability issues. Safe Harbor does protect the nurse from retaliation by an employer or contracted entity for whom the nurse performs nursing services. There is no expiration of the protection against retaliatory actions such as demotion, forced change of shifts, pay cut, or other retaliatory action against the nurse.

### (8) When Can a Smaller Workgroup of the Nursing Peer Review Committee be utilized?

A smaller workgroup of the nursing peer review committee may be used in either Safe Harbor or Incident-Based nursing peer review. The nurse involved in either type of peer review must agree to the use of the smaller workgroup. The nurse does not give up his/her right to review by the full peer review committee just because they initially agree to the smaller work group. As stated in the rule, the work group must be made up of members of the peer review committee, and must follow the same time lines, due process steps, and other procedures that apply to the full nursing peer review committee.

The peer review rules do not address use of a smaller work group of peer review in the event a nurse was terminated for practice related reasons. When a report to the BON is mandated under NPA 301.405(b), peer review is conducted solely to look for the existence of external factors that may have impacted the nurse's actions. Since neither the statute or board rules specifically allow or prohibit the use of the smaller work group for this purpose, facility policy and procedure on nursing peer review would need to address if this is an option for peer review under NPA 301.405(c).

**(9) Must the recommendations made by the SHPR Committee be followed by the CNO/Nurse Administrator? [NPR §303.005(d); rule 217.20(j)(4)(A)]**

NPR law §303.005(d) requires the employer/nurse manager to consider the decision of the SHPR Committee "in any decision to discipline the nurse." The "non-binding" provision in this statute means that if the CNO/Nurse Administrator believes the SHPR was conducted in "bad faith," or otherwise made an incorrect determination, the CNO/Administrator must document his/her rationale for disagreeing with the SHPR Committee determination, and this must be retained with the SHPR records. In addition, if the CNO/Nurse Administrator believes the SHPR was done in bad faith, he/she has a duty to report the nurses who participated on the PRC to the BON [see rule 217.20(j)(4)(C)].

The BON encourages CNOs/Nurse Administrators to remember that each nurse has a duty to advocate for patient/client safety. This is expressed in rule 217.11(1)(B) and explained in Position Statement 15.14 Duty of a Nurse in Any Setting. Both of these documents are located on the BON web page in multiple areas, but most easily found under the "Nursing Practice" link, and then under "Scope of Practice." Another document located in this section of the web page is the BON's Six-Step Decision-Making Model for Determining Nursing Scope of Practice. Step 3 asks if there is nursing literature, research, or guidance documents from national specialty nursing organizations related to the nursing issue in question. National patient safety organizations, such as the Institute for Safe Medication Practices, would also be applicable with regard to "best practices" in a given area of nursing and patient safety. Safe Harbor peer review can be an opportunity to take stock of how nursing and support departments surrounding nursing are organized, and how safe patient care is helped or hindered by those systems.

**If you have additional questions regarding Peer Review, see Nursing Peer Review (TOC) Chapter 303 and BON Rules 217.19 and 217.20**

Send questions and comments to: webmaster@bon.state.tx.us

# Internal Peer Review— Nurturing the Next Generation of Nursing Scholars for Evidence-Based Practice

*Courtesy of Porter Adventist Hospital,*
*Evidence-Based Practice Council*

CYNTHIA A. OSTER, PhD, MBA, APRN, CNS, ANP (CHAIR)
CAROL ALEXANDER, RN, MS
KATHLEEN BRADLEY, RN, MSN, NE-BC
SHERI CLARK, RN, BSN
JASON DiGREGORIO, DNP, RN, FNP
LAVONE HASTINGS, RN-BC, BSN, MMGT
CAROLYN LANNING, RN, BSN
RICHARD MAXWELL, RN, MLS
CLANCY MEYERS, MHA, EMT-P
SHARON PAPPAS, RN, PhD, NEA-BC
APRIL ROMERO, RN
RYAN STICE, PharmD

Internal peer review is a process to ensure that abstracts, posters, and podium presentations represent best scholarship prior to external dissemination. Peer review is an integral part of professional nursing practice that traditionally involves licensed personnel evaluating one another (Pederson, Crabtree, & Ortiz-Tomei, 2004). Scholarly journals use a peer review process when determining whether a manuscript should be accepted for publication (Miracle, 2008). Internal peer review is the process that professional nurses at Porter Adventist Hospital use to ensure that abstracts, posters, and podium presentations that will be disseminated for external presentation represent best scholarship.

This best practice is an innovative peer review process conducted in the Porter Adventist Hospital Evidence-Based Practice Council. The intent of internal peer review in this setting is to help nurses or other clinical authors achieve and maintain credibility by identifying errors, preserving scientific rigor, and reducing the potential for bias. The Evidenced-Based Practice (EBP) Council is an interdisciplinary council composed of both clinical and nonclinical professionals. Membership is decided by a passion for EBP and research. All levels of the nursing division, from staff nurses to chief nursing officers, hold membership and participate in the peer review process.

The EBP Council has been the venue for the conduct of internal peer reviews since 2007. One of the initial goals identified by the council was the advancement of nursing science. The council recognized the current hospital environment promoted quality improvement and EBP projects; however, nurses or other clinical staff and leaders lacked the knowledge or guidance on how to publicize or present improvements outside the hospital. Thus, the council established a strategic goal to increase the number of evidence-based projects externally disseminated through abstract submissions to regional and national conferences. Peer review was the avenue selected to ensure that these abstracts were the best scholarship and had the best opportunity for acceptance.

Peer review is a standing agenda item for council meetings. Professional clinical staff contacts the council chair or any council member to submit a project for review. Reviews are conducted in a timely manner and suggestions to the author are provided. Reviews are conducted during council meeting time, as well as virtually via e-mail and conference calls. The use of technology enables clinicians to incorporate peer review recommendations in a timely manner even though the council may not be in session (see Table 1).

Council members are expected to be fair, unbiased, and avoid harsh or demeaning comments throughout the peer review process. The intent of the internal peer review process is to be constructive and to support professional development. Abstracts are reviewed for clarity, guideline adherence, and scholarship.

A key component to peer review is coaching for improved scholarship. Coaching enables creative problem solving in a positive constructive environment (Kowalski & Casper, 2007).

Clinical staff has demonstrated a willingness to write and submit abstracts with the collaboration of a coach. Coaching from members of the EBP Council has occurred through one-on-one interaction, as well as through workshops sponsored by the EBP Council. Members of the council provide peer review during experiential learning sessions designed to teach participants how to write a scholarly abstract. These initial workshops spawned staff requests for coaching on how to do a podium or poster presentation. The outcome of these workshops was a greater number of abstracts submitted to regional and

**Table 1.  Porter Adventist Hospital EBP Council: Peer Review Algorithm**

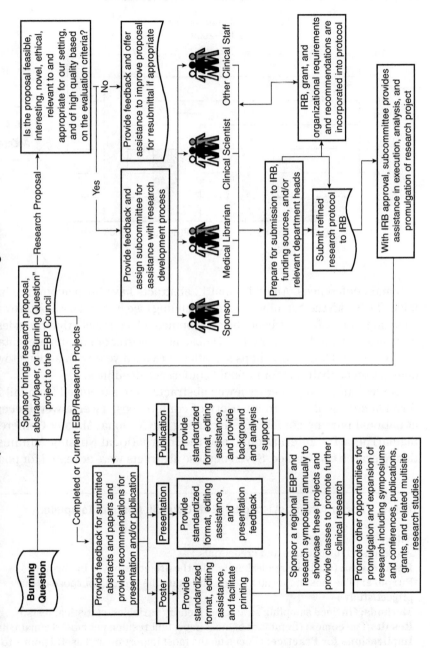

**Figure 1.    Growth of abstract submission and acceptance.**

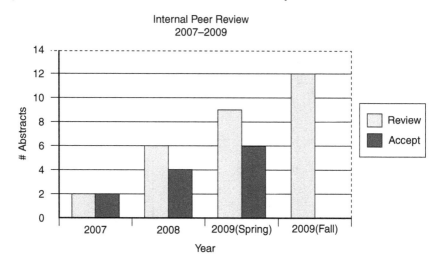

national conferences. An additional 12 abstracts have been submitted in the fall of 2009 with the outcome currently pending (see Figure 1). An outgrowth of coaching workshops has been the development of a template that provides the foundation to build an abstract and subsequent poster or podium presentation (see Table 2). These workshops are offered twice a year with a focus toward completion of abstracts for regional conference deadlines.

Sixteen internally peer-reviewed abstracts were submitted from fall 2006 through spring of 2009 to a variety of conferences. Twelve were accepted at national nursing conferences including the National Magnet Conference, Sigma Theta Tau International, and the International Nursing Administration Research Conference. Seven of these abstracts were accepted for podium

**Table 2.    Porter Adventist Hospital, EBP Council, Abstract Template.**

**Title:**
**Author(s):** (Include title and credentials.)
**Background:** (Grab the reader! State why the project/study is important.)
**Purpose:** (The most important statement! State the primary purpose of the project/study.)
**Methods:** (Include sampling strategies: identify variables, statistical tests.)
**Results/Outcomes:** (Summary of most important results; put most dramatic first.)
**Implications for Practice:** (Focus on the most important and useful points to the practice.)

**Figure 2.    Conference abstract acceptance.**

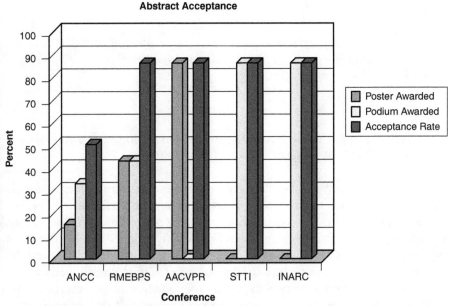

Abstract Acceptance

ANCC = American Nurses Credentialing Center National Magnet Conference
RMEBPS = Rocky Mountain EBP Symposium
AACVPR = American Association of Cardiovascular/Pulmonary Rehabilitation
STTI = Sigma Theta Tau International 20th International Nursing Research Congress
INARC = International Nursing Administration Research Conference

presentations whereas the other five were accepted for poster presentations (see Figure 2).

Submitting abstracts to conferences does not guarantee that the abstracts will be accepted. Factors that potentially increase the possibility of acceptance are the focus of peer review. One of these factors is how the authors title abstracts. Prior to implementation of the internal peer review process, a member of the EBP Council submitted an abstract electronically to a national conference. The abstract file was returned to the author unopened. The title did not properly reflect the focus of the conference. Peer review through the EBP Council has provided authors with constructive critique to increase the probability of abstracts submitted electronically to be opened and read by conference reviewers. Staff are coached in developing titles that are concise and descriptive of what is in the abstract. In addition, key words in the title describe the specific topic and subject matter with consideration of the proposed conference focus.

The following is an example of changing the title of an abstract after an internal peer review.

Before:

*"Commitment of Staff and Physicians to Improving Joint Replacement Patients' Safety by Reducing Falls Utilizing Specific Data Sources to Influence Nursing and Medical Practice"*

After:

*"Data Analysis: The Muscle Behind an Interdisciplinary Approach to Improving Safety for Joint Replacement Patients"*

Subsequent to acceptance of an abstract for presentation at a conference, the EBP Council continues to offer peer review as a resource to clinical staff in preparation for poster or podium presentations. Poster presenters bring examples of the poster to the EBP Council meetings. Posters are critiqued for effective visual elements (Keely, 2004). Examples of peer review focus include formatting, references, and placement of pictures and graphs. In addition, the council member with the most expertise serves as a resource to facilitate understanding and readability of content. This allows members of the council to assume leadership roles in areas of expertise and to serve as coaches to guide colleagues. Posters undergo a series of transformation during the internal peer review process (see Figures 3 and 4). Logistically, coaching can take place during a meeting or by e-mail. From the first draft of a poster through the final draft, the entire council is available for input and feedback. Peer review is expected to be creative, unbiased, and timely, not harsh in nature. Results of this process are encouraging.

Peer review can greatly influence the flavor of a podium presentation. Specifically, podium presentations are evaluated for clarity and style (Happell, 2009). Presenters are able to practice presentations before an audience intent on coaching and providing support. In addition, the interdisciplinary membership provides peer review through a variety of professional perspectives. The question-and-answer peer review session helps to prepare the authors for diverse questions at a conference. This process serves as a confidence booster and assists in identification and minimization of bias.

One example of internal peer review for presenters impacting a podium presentation is relayed in this testimonial from Kathleen Bradley, RN, MSN, NE-BC:

> After getting accepted for a podium presentation, I had the opportunity of presenting an evidenced-based management project of the float pool redesign and the subsequent financial impact on contract labor usage. The presentation had

# Figure 3. Poster version 1: Hypoglycemia – Let's Prevent and Treat It Right!

Porter Adventist Hospital
*Centura Health.*

## "Hypoglycemia – Let's Prevent It and Treat It Right!"

Dorcas A. Kipp RN, BSN, CDE, James Chappell MD, FACE, Robert Serravo PharmD, Cynthia A. Oster, PHD, MBA, RN, CNS, ANP

A Picture or a Map would be a nice addition here. Delete this textbox and add a graphic.

### Introduction

Fear of hypoglycemia has been found to be the primary limiting factor in the management of patient with diabetes. It was of utmost concern that we put systems in place that would limit hypoglycemia risk before intensifying blood glucose control. We focused on evidence based protocols for preventing and reducing hypoglycemia.

### Materials and Methods

Although we had implemented numerous protocols and procedures for preventing hypoglycemia, we were unable to quantify that our changes had actually created a safer environment for our patients. Random chart audits found incomplete documentation, and staff were not readily filing hypoglycemia occurrence reports. Risk management supported our request by serving as the centralized location for receiving these as well as all other occurrence reports. CDE initiated staff education on nursing units in 9/2007, using visual aids to help nursing staff better understand insulin action (fig 1), clarify how to use Hypoglycemia Occurrence Reporting Tool, and to effectively use the Hypoglycemia Treatment Protocol. Changes were implemented in the EMR that promoted better documentation of the hypoglycemic event. In addition, the hospital decided to purchase the RALS TGCM software which expanded our ability to evaluate both past and present BG trends and hypoglycemia occurrences.

There will be space here for a picture below the text

Another Figure

### Results

Sometimes people will just put bullets with short sentences, instead of lots of text. (In that case, make the text even bigger)

- Incidence of hypoglycemia was reduced from 5% of all POCT tests done in 2004 to only 2.5% of all POCT tests done in 2007

- ——% of episodes were treated per protocol

- ——% of all episodes were documented in the EMR correctly after re-education of staff

- Reduction in hypoglycemia resulted in estimated cost savings of $——— per year

### Abstract

**Background:** Observed inconsistency in treatment of hypoglycemia. Physicians reported that patients who had been treated for hypoglycemia frequently suffered rebound hyperglycemia. Review of American Diabetes Association National Standards for Care of the Hospitalized Patient and Practical Management of Inpatient Hyperglycemia by Hirsch, Braithwaite and Verderese clarified the need to standardize and upgrade treatment protocol. CDE worked with nursing and endocrinology to implement an evidence based protocol which was implemented in 3/2005. However, chart review in 3/2007 shows we still have a problem with documentation of proper treatment. Also, we are unable to quantify the numbers of episodes that occur in our institution. Attempted without success to implement a voluntary reporting tool in an effort to track volume trends in treatment, and effect of the protocol. We were unable to determine if hypoglycemia episodes are decreasing or if they are properly treated.

**Purpose:** To prevent hypoglycemic events and properly treat those events that occur.

**Methods:** Review of literature to learn how hypoglycemia is tracked in other institutions resulted in limited information. No successful tracking methods have been reported. New JACHO guidelines for inpatient management of hyperglycemia require this type of tracking for the purpose of understanding trends and improving the safety of hospitalized patients with diabetes. A multidisciplinary approach for prevention, treatment and tracking was implemented. In 9/2007 we implemented staff re-education to improve understanding of who is at risk for hypoglycemia so that if possible it can be prevented. CDE offered multiple classes on each nursing unit. The protocol title was clarified to include the word "prevention." Guidelines for using the protocol were clarified. Risk Management implemented a mandatory reporting tool. Our laboratory now has the ability to compile reports of Point of Care Tests, and can provide data on actual blood glucose results within the hospital which will help us track the trends in blood glucose data and quantify hypoglycemic events. We will use this data to give nursing staff feedback about improved glycemic control on their unit.

**Results/outcomes:** As hypoglycemia prevention and treatment increased, staff requested more information about diabetes care. Since June 2006, educational seminars have been offered to nursing staff. The focus of the seminar was to disseminate evidence from the literature for glycemic control in the hospital. In addition we have taught about insulin action, carbohydrate counting and tight control of blood glucose during illness. The protocol has been discussed at each seminar, as well as at new employee orientation, and new grad class. Pharmacists created a "Hypoglycemia Treatment Kit" in Pyxis (fig.2), that makes each of the treatment options readily available. Nutrition Services modified the hospital menu to include carbohydrate grams on all menu selections. RALS software shows decline in episodes of hypoglycemia by ——%. Audit of the EMR shows ——% treated per protocol, and ——% documented correctly.

**Implications for Practice:** Using research done by others, we recognized that our care of the hypoglycemic patient was not acceptable. We recognized that our nursing staff all had different backgrounds, and not all were used to treating hypoglycemia in a scientific manner. We recognized that we needed a protocol that was easy to use and that met the various needs of the hospitalized patient. This one change led to numerous other changes in the way we treat patients with diabetes.

### Discussion and Conclusions

This can be two separate sections (if you really want to highlight some conclusions) or a combo section.

### Literature Cited

Famous Scientist. 1999. Important literature. Important Journal 12:13-17.
Famous Scientist. 1999. Important literature. Important Journal 12:13-17.

### Acknowledgments

Research Monitor:

Funding: Project IBS-CORE Undergraduate Research Fellowship, provided by a grant from the Howard Hughes Medical Institute to the University of Montana.

**Figure 4.   Poster version 10: Hypoglycemia – Let's Prevent and Treat It Right!**

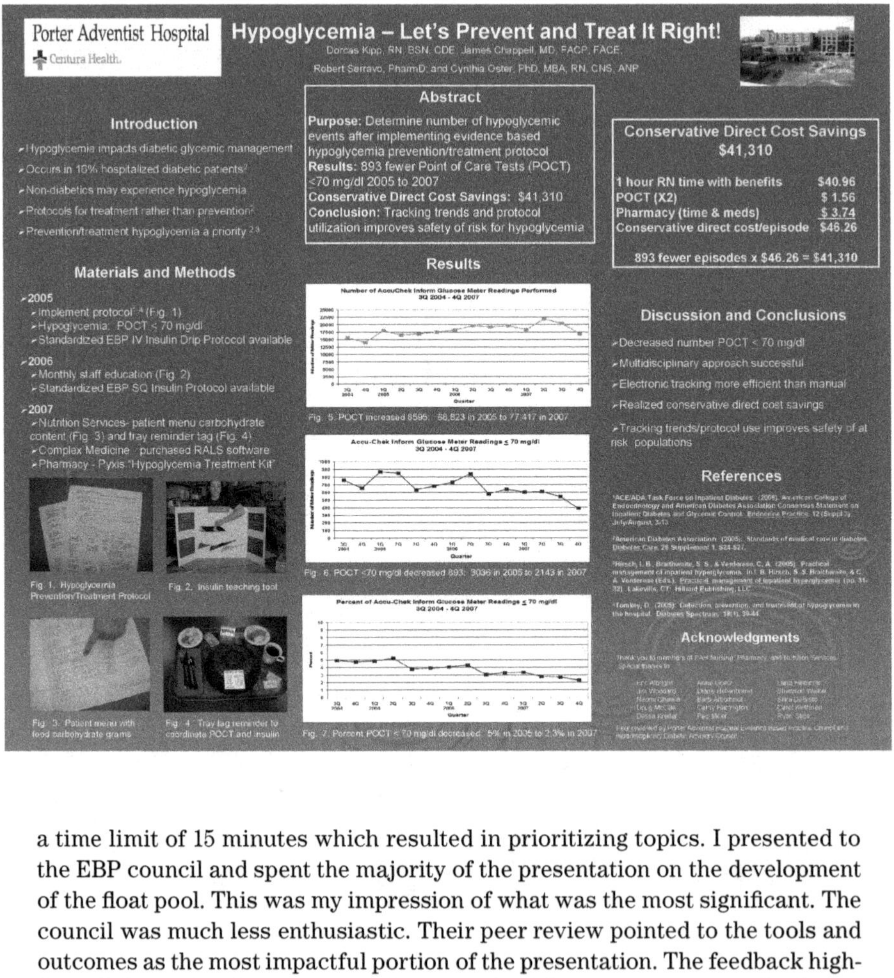

a time limit of 15 minutes which resulted in prioritizing topics. I presented to the EBP council and spent the majority of the presentation on the development of the float pool. This was my impression of what was the most significant. The council was much less enthusiastic. Their peer review pointed to the tools and outcomes as the most impactful portion of the presentation. The feedback highlighted the need to focus more on the strength of the outcomes versus the design of the project. The resulting presentation given at the conference was targeted at the tools, outcomes and impact for replication.

The EBP Council also serves as an entry point for future nursing scientists. Research proposals undergo internal peer review prior to the Institutional Review Board (IRB) submission. Internal peer review provides the novice researcher assistance with protocol development and IRB navigation.

In order to nurture our scholars and to prepare the next generation for the promotion of nursing science, the EBP Council sponsors an annual regional

EBP and research conference. The EBP Council has seen a tremendous growth in nursing science, as well as integration of interdisciplinary research and EBP projects. The council has exceeded the initial goal established when internal peer review was introduced. The initial goal has been expanded to include nurturing the next generation of nursing scholars beyond the walls of Porter Adventist Hospital to include scholars within the 12 hospital systems of Centura Health.

The expanded focus will include interdisciplinary collaboration and mentoring relationships among council members, clinical nurses, and other clinical staff throughout the 12 hospitals of Centura Health. The EBP Council plans to expand membership to include interdisciplinary membership from sister facilities. The concept of internal peer review provides the foundation for growth and nurturance of the next generation of scholars for the advancement of EBP at each individual facility and also throughout the corporation.

Nurturing the next generation of nursing scholars is imperative in order to contribute to the knowledge base that is foundational to the discipline of nursing. Internal peer review is a strategy that achieves and maintains scholarly credibility by identifying errors, preserving scientific rigor, and reducing bias. Interdisciplinary collaboration and mentoring relationships between council members and staff nurses are established. Opportunities for teaching and coaching are designed to provide valuable feedback to budding scholars on all aspects of abstract writing and poster or podium presentation prior to external dissemination.

Nurse authors develop greater confidence in their writing and presentation skills following internal peer review. Through teaching and coaching, the next generation of scholars can develop the skill set needed to write a clear, concise, and compelling abstract. In addition, nurse authors can present a poster or deliver a podium presentation with confidence at regional and national conferences. Scholars can confidently stand with their poster while interacting with conference participants knowing that the poster has been critiqued for visual effectiveness and accuracy. In addition, the internal peer review process helps to minimize the impact of nervousness that can occur prior to or during a podium presentation. Nurse scholars are poised during a podium presentation as the internal peer review process has validated the content, audiovisuals, and their presentation style. Internal peer review prior to external dissemination enables the next generation of scholars to be at ease when presenting their work.

## REFERENCES

Happell, B. (2009). Presenting with precision: Preparing and delivering a polished conference presentation. *Nurse Researcher, 16*(3), 45–56.

Keely, B. R. (2004). Planning and creating effective scientific posters. *The Journal of Continuing Education in Nursing, 35*(4), 182–185.

Kowalski, K., & Casper, C. (2007). The coaching process: An effective tool for professional development. *Nursing Administration Quarterly, 31*(2), 171–179.

Miracle, V. A. (2008). The peer review process. *Dimensions in Critical Care Nursing, 27*(2), 67–69.

Pederson, A., Crabtree, T., & Ortiz-Tomei, T. (2004). Implementation of the peer review council. *MEDSURG Nursing, 13*(3), 172–175.

# Description of Development of Nursing Case Review

Nursing Peer Review

**SUNY Downstate Medical Center**

**445 Lenox Road**

**Brooklyn, NY**

*Courtesy of SUNY Downstate Medical Center*

Nursing Peer Review based on actual or "near miss" adverse events or occurrences provides nurses with the opportunity to examine in-depth the relationship of nursing actions to patient outcomes. Kearney (2001) notes that professional responsibility and accountability involves upholding, developing, and critically analyzing quality standards and outcomes: As professionals, she says, nurses are responsible for nursing care outcomes (p.12). As Hunt (2008) noted, a nursing peer review forum facilitates, " in-depth, thoughtful examination of nursing practice, recognition of practice patterns, and determination of nursing action steps to mitigate patient problems" (p. 14).

Until a few years ago, if a patient-adverse event occurred, nursing review at SUNY Downstate Medical Center was conducted by nursing management personnel. Often an adverse-patient event would be referred to the nursing department only after physicians had reviewed the case and determined that nursing care was involved in the occurrence. This process began to change in 2004 when a new chief nursing officer (CNO) was appointed who envisioned staff nurses being active in all decision-making processes that affected clinical care of patients. With this new vision, an occurrence-based nursing peer review process was created. Nursing issues are addressed more thoroughly and nursing is better prepared for participation in the hospital root cause analysis process.

The nursing department sought to develop a consistent, effective, and impartial process to achieve true peer review. The first step was to define what we meant by peer review. We turned to the American Nurses Association (ANA) definition as cited in the Peer Review Guidelines:

> Peer review is an organized effort whereby practicing professionals review the quality and appropriateness of services ordered or performed by their professional peers. Peer Review in Nursing is the process by which practicing Registered Nurses systematically assess, monitor, and make judgments about the quality of nursing care provided by peers, as measured against professional standards of practice. (ANA, 1988)

A nursing peer review committee was formed, comprised of nursing representation from management, education, clinical practice, and performance improvement. Staff nurses are chosen from the unit involved, as well as similar units.

The Nursing Peer Review Committee conducts peer reviews based on established criteria. Any member of the nursing department may initiate the process as well as staff from other departments. Cases that are referred for peer review may include, but are not limited to:

- Events involving wrong patient, wrong procedure, wrong site;
- Errors of omission leading to death or serious injury;
- Failure to rescue leading to significant deterioration of patient's condition;
- Medication error with actual or potential serious harm, near death, or death;
- Falls with fracture or head injury;
- Any patient care situation that jeopardizes patient safety.

Prior to the committee convening, an investigation is conducted through review of the medical record and interviews with staff directly and indirectly involved (conducted by the nurse manager, the associate director of nursing PI, and/or a member of the hospital performance improvement department).

The peer review members use a consistent format for the discussion of each incident that includes:

- Description of the incident—involves brief history, medical, and nursing assessment noting any actual or potential nursing issues
- Review of staffing—may be quality or quantity; issues of experience, education, ratio of permanent staff to contracted personnel
- Communication breakdowns—among nurses, nurses and physicians, other departments;

- Equipment issues—whether or not equipment was involved, including working order and staff competency
- Medication—whether or not medication was involved; including patient monitoring, staff knowledge of the medication, medication administration;
- Clinical care standards—evidence-based standards related to this issue and compliance to same
- Patient factors—such as changes in condition, education, or cultural factors
- Physical layout—placement of patient on nursing unit
- Information management—availability of current comprehensive information to make appropriate assessments and care decisions
- Policies/procedures/protocols—which address the situation and compliance to same
- Literature review—clinical literature and/or patient safety literature
- Summary and conclusions—was the standard of nursing practice met?
- Plan of correction—if applicable, this may include both individual and systems-based recommendations

Each area is reviewed to determine if there was deviation from established standards of nursing practice. The peer review committee analyzes the incident to arrive at the nursing root cause(s). Root causes may be systems based, individual performance based, or both. Each case is scored for nursing root cause and for the documentation of nursing care (see Table 1). The score is used to help determine a plan of correction. A report of the committee's findings and recommended actions is prepared and submitted to the CNO and the nursing performance improvement and patient safety council. The council discusses the case and may suggest further recommendations to the plan of correction. Major discussion points are included in council minutes. Upon CNO and council approval, the report is forwarded to the hospital performance improvement department.

The journey from management-controlled investigations to bedside nurses peer-reviewing near misses and actual adverse events took several years. At first, staff were very hesitant to speak in front of other colleagues and management.

**Table 1. Nursing Peer Review Scoring Grid**

| Clinical Care (score all) | Documentation |
|---|---|
| 0—Care Appropriate | A—Exemplary |
| 1—System error/Error | B—Consistent |
| 2—Individual performance concern | C—Below standard |

Consistent encouragement was needed for staff nurses to openly discuss nursing practice issues and peer performance. Staff nurses were reassured that all discussions were confidential and that each individual's privacy was maintained. Some nursing leaders were defensive and protective of territory in the beginning stages. Understanding the role that systems play in errors was accomplished through consistent education and thorough discussion of each case. Gradually, fears of recrimination lessened and trust in the process increased.

The following case study illustrates the process we follow for our nursing peer reviews.

*Case Study: Investigating A Near-Miss Medication Incident*

- Description of Incident—This patient was a 69-year-old male who presented to the emergency department with chief complaints of constipation, nausea, and vomiting for 2 days. The patient was admitted to one of our critical care units for anemia in the presence of bright red rectal bleeding and partial small bowel obstruction. During his course in the critical care unit, the lab called to report an elevated magnesium level. The nurse assigned to the patient recorded the values and notified the physician. A medication error occurred when the physician ordered a dose of magnesium and the nurse administered the dose. There was no adverse patient occurrence.
- Staffing—A review of the staffing pattern indicated that the established nurse–patient ratio and staff mix was in place. All staff were experienced full-time nurses with one long-term contract nurse. It was noted that all nurses had current competencies on file, including the contract nurse who had worked in this particular unit for over 1 year.
- Communication—There were deficits in communication between nurse and physician. The correct procedure was followed for "Write Down–Read Back" by the nurse who entered the results on the correct form in the chart, but the results were verbally told to the physician. Shortly after, the nurse realized her mistake and notified the physician and nursing leadership.
- Equipment—The medication was taken from the automatic dispensing unit (ADU). The ADU high alert for magnesium was greater than the patient's level and thus there was no alert generated.
- Medication—During the initial interview with the nurse prior to the peer review committee being convened, a knowledge deficit of electrolyte values was identified.
- Clinical Issues—This was determined to be a very complex patient with many comorbidities but there were no clinical issues that directly impacted this incident.

- Information management—Our hospital is in the process of implementing an electronic medical record but at the time of this incident, all entries were manually created. There was difficulty reading some of the entries of nurses and physicians, but this was not determined to be a factor. This review did uncover a problem in retrieving computerized patient laboratory information. Long-term contract nurses at the time of this incident did not have access to computerized laboratory results.
- Policies and procedures—The peer review committee determined that this incident was not related to lack of appropriate policies or procedures.
- Literature review—One of the most pertinent articles reviewed was from the *Nurse Advise-ERR*: Preventing Magnesium Toxicity in Obstetrics (ISMP Medication Safety Alert, 2006). This article addresses accidental overdose of magnesium in the obstetrics units. The article cites several examples of accidental overdose. Although the situations described are not the same as the case presented, similar contributing factors such as hurried hand-off report, high-unit acuity, and lack of magnesium toxicity assessment were noted.
- Summary and conclusions—A medication error occurred that was considered a near miss. The error did not have an adverse impact on patient outcome but could have potentially harmed the patient. This near-miss event emphasized opportunities for improvement in individual performance and systems. On the individual level, additional education and competence assessment was provided for this practitioner. On the systems level, several changes were implemented. Long-term contract staff were given computer access equal to permanent staff following training and competency assessment. This enabled safer communication among all providers and quicker access to patient information. An opportunity to improve safety through the ADU was also identified. After this incident, the pharmacy reset the high and low alert values for several key electrolytes. This now alerts the practitioner before levels reach a life-threatening level.

The Nursing Peer Review Process at our hospital has enabled professional nurses to examine nursing issues in a safe and nonpunitive environment. As a result of the peer review process, changes have been made to several medication processes as well as other policies and procedures. Our next step is to update our orientation program to provide the opportunity for all new nurses to observe a peer review during their orientation. Participation of frontline nurses, who are in the best position to describe actual bedside practice patterns, significantly contributes to the realistic analysis of nursing practice issues and the development of improved nursing care processes.

## REFERENCES

American Nurses Association. (1988). Peer review guidelines. *American Nurses Association Publications*, *i-iv*, 1–14.

Hunt, V. (2008). Implementing a nursing peer review process, *Forum*, *26*, 2, 14–15. Available at: www.rmf.harvard.edu/files/documents/Forum_V26N2-hunt.pdf. Accessed January 21, 2010.

ISMP Medication Safety Alert. (2006). Preventing magnesium toxicity in obstetrics. *Nurse Advise-ERR*, *4*(6), 1–2.

Kearney, R. (2001). *Advancing your career: Concepts of professional nursing* (2nd ed.). Philadelphia, PA: F. A. Davis.

# Nursing Peer Case Review

*Courtesy of OSF Rockford, Rockford, IL*

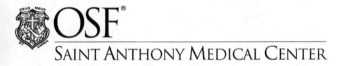

### SAINT ANTHONY MEDICAL CENTER

| TITLE:<br>NURSING PEER CASE REVIEW | POLICY NUMBER:<br>PI-NUR-929 |
|---|---|
| **ORIGINAL DATE:** March 2008 | **REVISION DATE:** |
| **REVIEW DATE:** March 2011 | **REVIEWED BY:**<br>Executive Coordinating Council &<br>Nursing Practice Council |
| **APPROVAL SIGNATURE:** | |

## GENERAL

*"Standards of nursing practice provide a means for measuring the quality of nursing care a client receives. Each nurse is responsible for interpreting and implementing the standards of nursing practice."*
*(ANA Peer Review Guidelines, 1983, p. 3)*

*"Peer review implies that the nursing care delivered by a group of nurses or an individual nurse is evaluated by individuals of the same rank or standing according to established standards of practice."*
*(ANA Peer Review Guidelines, 1983, p. 3)*

*"As the professional association for nursing, ANA has a responsibility to the public and its members to facilitate the development of a quality assurance system including peer review."*
*(ANA Peer Review Guidelines, 1983, p. 2)*

## PURPOSE

Nursing peer case review is designed to provide a process by which nurses systematically assess and evaluate the quality of nursing care provided by peers, as measured against professional standards of practice in climate of collegial problem solving and a continuous learning environment. The results of such assessments are used to promote safe, high quality care.

The purpose of nursing peer case review is to maintain standards of nursing practice in a non-punitive manner while encouraging peer support in order to improve patient care. Peer case review provides an opportunity for staff to be evaluated by peers knowledgeable of their job duties, scope of practice, and responsibilities. The goals of peer case review are to:

- Improve patient outcomes
- Identify learning opportunities
- Promote nursing excellence
- Enhance nursing image and professionalism
- Support and encourage nurse autonomy and accountability
- Facilitate a sensitive and caring peer review interaction

The Executive Coordinating Council is responsible for creating, evaluating, and overseeing the nursing peer case review process. The Nursing Practice Council (NPC) is responsible for implementing and providing input regarding the nursing peer case review process.

## DEFINITIONS

### Nursing Staff

All licensed hospital and contract nursing personnel (RNs and LPNs) delivering care to patients at OSF Saint Anthony Medical Center (SAMC).

### Nursing Peer Case Review

Nursing peer case review is the process by which nurses systematically assess and make recommendations about the quality and appropriateness of nursing care provided by their peers. Standards of practice are defined by the Illinois Nurse Practice Act and Rules, the American Nurses Association Scope and Standards of Practice, and the appropriate nursing specialty organizations. The Nursing Practice Council (NPC) will make recommendations that facilitate a nurse's successful practice of high quality, competent nursing care. All nursing peer case review is conducted internally at OSF Saint Anthony Medical Center.

Nursing peer case review is conducted using multiple sources of information, including the review of individual cases, the review of aggregate data for compliance, clinical standards, and the use of rates compared against established benchmarks or norms when applicable. Cases are selected for review that relate to quality of care, technical errors, documentation, risk issues, complaints, and other sources.

The evaluation of a case is based on generally recognized professional standards of care. This peer case review process provides nurses with feedback for personal improvement or confirmation of personal achievement related to the effectiveness of their nursing, technical, ethical, and interpersonal skills in providing patient care.

### Initial Case Review

A member of the Quality Care Management Division (QCM nurse, Patient Safety Officer, Risk Manager, Clinical Data Analyst), as a designee of NPC, conducts the initial case review using the OSF SAMC Nursing Peer Case Review Form. If initial review meets designated requirements, the case is then referred on to the specialty case reviewer.

### Specialty Case Reviewer

A specialty case reviewer designated by NPC is an RN, in good standing, who conducts an evaluation once the initial reviewer refers the case. This RN is an Advanced Practice Nurse (APN) or a nurse on staff who holds a specialty certification or clinical ladder 4 and/or masters prepared bedside nurse in the area of practice in which the case situation occurs.

### Peer Case Reviewer

The peer case reviewer reviews cases on behalf of the Nursing Practice Council, and may or may not be a member of the Nursing Practice Council. A peer case reviewer is a member of the nursing staff, in good standing, within the same nursing specialty if possible as the patient case under review. Opinions from another nursing specialty may be offered and considered regarding specific issues related to the management of the case under review. An individual functioning as a peer case reviewer will not have provided care for the patient whose case is under review; however, opinions and information may be obtained from participants that were involved in the patient's care.

### Conflict of Interest

A member of the nursing staff asked to perform nursing peer case review may have a conflict of interest if he or she might not be able to render an unbiased opinion due to either involvement in the patient's case or a relationship with the nurse(s) involved. It is the peer case reviewer's obligation to disclose the potential conflict. The Nursing Practice Council's responsibility is to determine whether the conflict would prevent the individual(s) from participating and the extent of that participation. Individuals determined to have a conflict may not be present during peer case review discussions or decisions, other than to provide requested information.

### Confidentiality

The Nursing Practice Council (NPC) functions in accordance with the requirements of the IL Nurse Practice Act when engaging in nursing peer case review. The NPC members participate in the review process in good faith with extensive protection against incurring civil liability because of their participation, as provided by the Illinois law, including, but not limited to, the Illinois Medical Studies Act.

- Nursing peer case review proceedings are confidential, and any communication made to the Nursing Practice Council including its designees during peer case review is privileged.
- A member, agent, or employee may not disclose or be required to disclose any communication made to the committee or a record or proceeding of the committee.
- A person who attends nursing peer case review proceedings may not disclose or be required to disclose:
  - Information acquired in connection with the proceedings
  - An opinion, recommendation, or evaluation of the council or a council member
- Members of the Nursing Practice Council and participants may not be questioned about their testimony or about their opinions formed as a result of the council proceedings.
- Nursing Practice Council members are required to protect the identity of patients as much as possible.

**POLICY**

1. The involved nurse(s) will receive appropriate feedback as indicated by the NPC.
2. The hospital will use the nursing peer case review results in its performance improvement activities as appropriate.
3. The hospital will keep nursing peer case reviews and other quality information concerning a nurse in a secure location. Nursing peer case review includes information related to:
   a. Performance data for dimensions of performance measured for an individual nurse
   b. The individual's role in sentinel events, significant incidents, or near misses
   c. Correspondence to the nurse regarding commendations, comments regarding performance or corrective action
   d. Nursing peer case review information is available only to authorized individuals who have a legitimate need to know this information to fulfill their duties with regards to quality control or other medical studies to reduce morbidity and mortality and improvement of patient care based on their responsibilities as hospital employee and according to hospital policy on access to information.
4. No copies of nursing peer case review documents will be created and distributed unless authorized by hospital policy.
5. The Nursing Practice Council will review the findings of individual(s) case review for a nurse(s) who exceed thresholds (see #6). The NPC determines whether further intensive review is needed to identify a potential pattern that impacts the provision of safe high quality care.
6. Thresholds for focused review include:
   a. Any single egregious case
   b. Within any 12 month period of time, any one of the following criteria:
      i. Three cases rated impact of care as major impact
      ii. Five cases rated impact of care as moderate impact
      iii. Five cases rated as having documentation concerns, regardless of impact of care
7. Nursing Peer case review is conducted by the NPC in a timely manner. The goal is for routine cases to be completed within 90 days from the date the case is identified or screened; complex cases are to be completed within 120 days. Exceptions may occur based on case complexity or reviewer availability.
8. Steps for sentinel events requiring nursing peer case review are in accordance with the Sentinel Event policy. Additional information (such as a literature search, second opinion, or external peer case review) may be necessary before making a decision on action. Under these

circumstances, the timelines may be extended after approval from the Executive Coordinating Council (ECC).

9. All nursing peer case review information is privileged and confidential in accordance with the hospital bylaws, state and federal laws and regulations pertaining to confidentiality and non-discoverability.

## PROCEDURE

1. Nursing peer case review is conducted by the NPC on an ongoing basis and reported for quality assurance purpose to the appropriate council, committee, or person for review and action.
2. Nursing peer review cases will be identified using the following sources:
   a. OSF SAMC departments or employees
   b. Nursing Practice Council
   c. Medical staff members
      i. Medical Staff Peer Review process, which identified cases for Nursing Peer Case Reviews, will be initiated in accordance with MS-MSS-04 Medical Staff Practice Evaluation and Peer Review policy
      ii. Referrals can include:
         1. Case review concerns
         2. Utilization concerns such as delay of discharge, prolonged length of stay, criteria not being met
         3. Care trends identified by any internal or external data source
         4. An unusual individual case or clinical pattern of care is identified during a quality review.
   d. Risk Management
   e. Patient Safety
      i. Cases identified for nursing peer case review via Occurrence or Near Miss will be initiated by the Vice President of Quality and Patient Safety, Patient Safety Officer, or designee and acts on behalf of the Quality/Patient Safety Council in accordance with AD-GN-21 Occurrence and Near Miss Process, Sentinel Event Reporting.
   f. Patients
   g. Families
   h. Payers
   i. State organizations
   j. Indicators as defined by the Shared Governance Councils or Subcouncils
   k. Patient satisfaction data
3. Cases selected for review include those related to:
   a. Quality of care (critical thinking)
   b. Technical errors

    c. Documentation

    d. Risk issues

    e. Complaints

    f. Other

4. Once a case has been identified for review, the OSF SAMC nursing peer case review process and time frames will be initiated and followed (see Appendix A—process flow chart).

5. The initial reviewer, as a designee of the NPC will complete the preliminary scoring for cases identified for nursing peer case review using the Nursing Peer Case Review Form.

6. If care is deemed appropriate, the NPC will process the scoring form and include the case in "no issue" cases reported to ECC.

    a. Nursing peer case reviews indicating appropriate nursing care by the initial reviewer are reported to the NPC for summary approval.

    b. If care is determined to be appropriate, the nurse will be informed of the decision by routine letter.

7. If issues are identified by the initial reviewer, the initial reviewer will contact the appropriate clinical nurse specialist/advanced practice nurse (APN) or specialty certified nurse designated by the NPC to act on behalf of the NPC within 1 week to complete the rating form.

    a. The initial review will provide the specialty reviewer a case summary and identify key issues.

    b. The specialty reviewer will complete the review within 2 weeks of obtaining the chart.

    c. If the specialty reviewer determines that issues do not exist and care was appropriate, the NPC will process the scoring form.

    d. If the specialty reviewer determines that issues do exist, the NPC will confirm the issues and a full review will take place.

8. Reviews indicating controversial nursing care are presented to the NPC by the specialty review for discussion and confirmation or change in preliminary scoring.

    a. If the NPC feels that care may be controversial, the NPC representative will contact the involved nurse to review key questions.

    b. The involved nurse(s) are informed of the key questions regarding the case and asked to respond.

    c. If care is determined to be controversial, involved nurse(s) are informed of the decision by nursing leadership.

9. If the results of peer case review indicate trends and a need for individual nurse action, the issue will be referred to the appropriate nursing manager/director for the appropriate human resource interventions. The manager/director will work with the individual nurse to create, implement, and evaluate a plan for positive outcome.

10. The specialty case reviewer and/or Nursing Practice Council will rate the case in the areas of patient outcomes, overall nursing care, effect on patient care, and nursing issue identification (see OSF SAMC Nursing Peer Case Review Form).
11. The specialty case reviewer and/or Nursing Practice Council may request additional information from the individuals or departments during the peer case review process.
12. Completed reviews will be submitted to the quality analyst by the specialty case reviewer and/or NPC chair to enter the case into the review tracking system.
13. The specialty case reviewer will discuss findings with staff members involved (if needed).
14. The aggregate information will be reported at least annually at the Nursing Executive Coordinating Council meeting.
15. The completed review forms are forwarded to the quality analyst for closure and trending.
16. The Chief Nursing Officer (CNO) will be notified of failure to respond to notification from the Nursing Practice Council. The CNO will follow up with the nurse manager and director requesting the required written explanation to be sent to the Nursing Practice Council.
17. The quality management department will enter the results of all final review findings into the database for tracking.
18. For cases with potential opportunities for improving system performance or potential issues with nursing care, the Nursing Practice Council will communicate the issue to the appropriate SAMC Department or committee.
19. Additional information (e.g., literature searches, second opinion, or external peer case review) may be necessary before making a decision or action. Under these circumstances, the time lines may be extended after approval from the Executive Coordinating Council.

## REFERENCES

### Statutory authority:

The above policy is based on the statutory authority of the Health Care Quality Improvement Act of 1986, 42 U.S.C. IIIOI, MEDICAL STUDIES ACT, Illinois Statute, chapter 735, ILCS 5/8-2101.

IL Nurse Practice Act and Rules. 2008

ANA *Peer Review Guidelines*, 1983, pages 2 and 3.

Revised 5/5/08, 6/17/08, 9/1/09

Account #_____    Discharge date _____

Date Reported _____    Nurse # _____

**Referral source**: Check the corresponding box

**Quality Division:**    ☐ **Q/CM Nurse**        ☐ **Clinical Data Analyst**

                       ☐ **Risk Management**    ☐ **Patient Safety Officer**

**Location of issue:** Check the corresponding box

☐ **ED**        ☐ **OR**  ☐ **PACU**  ☐ **ACC**      ☐ **Imaging**

☐ **Center for Cancer**  ☐ **ICU**  ☐ **Floor** _____  ☐ **Other** _____

**Review criteria/Referral issue:** _____

_____

**Case summary:** _____

_____

_____

_____

_____

_____

**Key issues for nurse reviewer:** _____

_____

_____

_____

_____

_____

_____

**To be completed by Specialty Case Reviewer**

**Nurse reviewer:** _____

                                    **Review date:** _____

|   |   | **Outcome: Check one** |   |   | **Effect on patient care: Check one** |
|---|---|---|---|---|---|
|   | 1 | No adverse outcome |   | 1 | Care not affected |
|   | 2 | Minor adverse outcome (complete recovery expected) |   | 2 | Increased monitoring/ observation (e.g., vital sign checks) |

| | 3 | Major adverse outcome (complete recovery **NOT** expected) |
| | 4 | Catastrophic adverse outcome (e.g., death) |

| | 3 | Additional treatment/ intervention (e.g., IV fluids) |
| | 4 | Life sustaining treatment/ intervention (e.g., CPR) |

| | | **Overall nursing care: Check one** |
|---|---|---|
| | 1 | Appropriate |
| | 2 | Controversial |
| | 3 | Inappropriate |
| | 0 | Reviewer uncertain, needs committee discussion |

| | | **Issue identification: Check all that apply** |
|---|---|---|
| | A | No issues with nursing care |
| | | **Nursing care issues** |
| | B | Critical thinking |
| | C | Assessment |
| | D | Technique/skills |
| | E | Knowledge |
| | F | Communication |
| | G | Planning |
| | H | Follow-up/follow-through |
| | I | Policy compliance |
| | J | Supervision (nursing student) |
| | O | Other: |

**Note:** If overall care = 1, **then** issue must = (A);
If overall care = 2, 3, or 0,
**then** issue must = (B) through (O)

If overall nursing care rated 2, 3, or 0, give a **brief description** of the basis for reviewer findings or concerns:

_____

_____

_____

_____

If overall nursing care rated 2, 3, or 0, **what questions** are to be addressed by the nurse or the council?

_____

_____

_____

_____

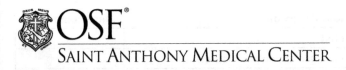

SAINT ANTHONY MEDICAL CENTER

| | | Nursing documentation: Check all that apply |
|---|---|---|
| | 1 | No issue with nursing documentation or nursing plan of care |
| | 2 | Documentation does not substantiate clinical course and treatment or plan of care |
| | 3 | Documentation not timely to communicate with other caregivers |
| | 4 | Documentation unreadable |
| | 9 | Other: |

**Documentation issue description:**

_____

_____

**Exemplary nominations:** ____ Nursing care ____ Nursing documentation
**Brief description** _____

_____

**Non-nursing care issues:** ____ Potential system or process issue
                                ____ Potential nursing care issue

**Issue description** _____

_____

---

**To Be Completed by Nursing Practice Council Reviewer**

Is nurse response needed? ____ Y ____N

**Nurse response:** ____ Discussion with chair ____ Letter
                       ____ Committee appearance

**Committee final scoring:**
Outcome: _____          Documentation: _____
Problem identification: _____          Overall nursing care _____

| Committee action: Check one | Date completed |
|---|---|
| No action warranted | |
| Nurse self-acknowledged action plan sufficient | |
| Educational letter to nurse sufficient | |
| Dept. manager discussion of informal improvement plan with nurse | |
| Dept. manager develops formal improvement plan with monitoring | |
| Refer to nursing leadership for formal corrective action | |

___ System problem identified—forward to VP of Quality/Patient Safety Council

Date sent _____          Date response _____

Describe system issue _____
_____
_____

___ Nursing standards issue—forward to nursing leadership

Date sent _____          Date response _____

Describe nursing concern _____
_____
_____

___ Potential physician issue—forward to medical staff

Date sent _____

_____

_____
Nursing Practice Council Chair

7/9/2008; Revised 10/23/08 (added Plan of Care to nursing documentation section)

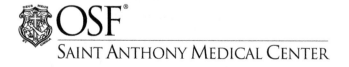

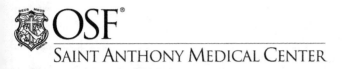

**Nursing Peer Review Executive Summary**                    **Date:**

| **1. Peer Review Summary**: Total Number of cases reviewed: | | | | |
|---|---|---|---|---|
| Number of Cases Referred from: | | | | |
| ED | | | Center for Cancer Care | |
| OR | | | ICU | |
| PACU | | | Floor | |
| ACC | | | Other | |
| IMAGING | | | | |

| **2. Outcomes:** | |
|---|---|
| **No Impact** on patient outcome | |
| **Minimal Impact**: Contributed to or resulted in temporary harm to the patient and required intervention | |
| **Moderate Impact**: Contributed to or resulted in temporary harm to the patient and required initial or prolonged hospitalization | |
| **Major Impact**: Contributed to or resulted in permanent patient harm | |
| **Major Impact**: Contributed to a near death event or required intensive medical care (intervention to sustain life) | |
| **Severe Impact**: Contributed to the patient's death | |
| **Impact cannot be accurately determined**: =X | |

| **3. Overall Nursing Care** | |
|---|---|
| Appropriate | |
| Controversial | |
| Inappropriate | |
| Reviewer uncertain, needs committee discussion | |

| **4. Effects on Patient Care** | |
|---|---|
| Care Not Affected | |
| Increased monitoring/observation (e.g., vital signs) | |
| Additional treatment/intervention (e.g., IV fluids) | |
| Life sustaining treatment/intervention (e.g., CPR) | |

| 5. Nursing Documentation | |
|---|---|
| No issue with nursing documentation | |
| Documentation does not substantiate clinical course and treatment | |
| Documentation not timely to communicate with other caregivers | |
| Documentation unreadable | |
| Other: | |
| **6. Issue Identification** | |
| No issues | |
| Critical thinking | |
| Assessment | |
| Technique/skills | |
| Knowledge | |
| Communication | |
| Planning | |
| Follow-up/follow-through | |
| Policy compliance | |
| Supervision (nursing student) | |
| Other: | |
| **7. Committee Action** | |
| No action warranted | |
| Nurse self-acknowledged action plan sufficient | |
| Educational offering - describe | |
| Individual counseling and discussion by: | |
| Formulation of new policy or procedure – referred to: | |
| System opportunity - Refer to Quality Patient Safety Council | |
| Medical Staff opportunity – refer to medical staff | |
| Refer to nursing manager for formal corrective action such as department manager develops formal improvement plan with monitoring | |
| Nursing practice standards issue—forward to nursing manager | |
| Other – describe: | |

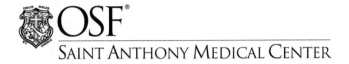

SAINT ANTHONY MEDICAL CENTER

## ROCKFORD, ILLINOIS
## CONFIDENTIALITY OF PEER REVIEW ACTIVITIES

As an OSF Saint Anthony Medical Center employed nurse who is involved in the evaluation and improvement of the quality of patient care rendered at OSF Saint Anthony Medical Center (i.e. Executive Coordinating Council, Nursing Practice Council, individual nurse assisting a peer review committee, or allied health professional participating in the credentialing review process), are provided with, and have access to, very sensitive and confidential information regarding nursing and other practitioner credentialing, quality improvement, and peer review activities.

It is of vital importance that all such information, and any and all discussions and deliberations regarding the same, be maintained in strict confidence. No disclosures of such confidential information may be made outside of appropriate meetings, except in the following very limited circumstances: when the disclosures are to another authorized employee of the hospital and are for the purpose of conducting peer review. A breach of this confidentiality may compromise the interests of OSF Saint Anthony Medical Center, nursing staff and its Medical Staff. Therefore, a breach of confidentiality may result in:

1. Dismissal from the committee, including peer review assignments;
2. Loss of available legal protections (including loss of indemnification for any litigation costs and expenses);
3. Disciplinary action as deemed appropriate by the Positive Discipline policy (Human Resources 601).

By signing below I acknowledge that I have received and read this document.

_____                    _____

Date                                              Signature


                                                  _____

                                                  Printed Name

August 12, 2008
(DATE)

RN NAME
UNIT

Dear XXX:
As you are aware, OSF Saint Anthony Medical Center is now conducting Nursing Peer Case Review. Recently one of your cases was evaluated by the Nursing Practice Council. On behalf of the Nursing Community of Caregivers, we would like to acknowledge you for your exemplary care and documentation with this patient.

We appreciate your dedication to our patients and continued pursuit of nursing excellence. Through the opportunity to review such cases we gain greater insight and appreciation for the role nurses play in providing excellent patient care.

Warm regards,


Stephanie Feltes, BSN, RN, TNS
Nursing Practice Council Chair


Paula Carynski, MS, RN, NEA-BC
Chief Nursing Officer

# *Index*

Note: Page numbers followed by *t* or *f* indicate material in tables or figures, respectively.

CPSIA information can be obtained
at www.ICGtesting.com
Printed in the USA
FSHW011710110719
59827FS